Homoeopathic Leaders in Pneumonia

By

Drs. A. and D. T. Pulford

Members of the International Hahnemannian Association

B. JAIN PUBLISHERS (P) Ltd.
NEW DELHI—110055

Price : Rs. 12.00

Reptint Edition : 1993

Published by :
B. Jain Publishers Pvt. Ltd.
1921, Street No. 10, Chuna Mandi
Paharganj, New Delhi - 110 055 (INDIA)

Printed at :
J.J. Offset Printers
Kishan Kunj, Delhi - 110 092

ISBN 81-7021-246-4
BOOK CODE B-2429

To
The Memories of
Hahnemann, Boenninghausen, Hering and Kent,
without whose efforts this little Monograph could not have been written and—

To
All True Homoeopaths Everywhere—
this little Monograph is most respectfully Dedicated.

The Authors.

PREFACE

No apology is needed for the birth of this little Monograph, the appalling mortality among pneumonia patients attests the demand for just such an one.

It has been stated, and we have every reason to believe truly, that fully 80% of all pneumonia cases would get well without any medical interference whatever, under proper nursing, so that any system or method of medical healing that cannot lower the death-rate to less than 20% would seem rather a menace than a blessing to pneumonia patients.

After treating 242 cases of pneumonia, of ALL types and degrees of severity, some coming directly from and others having been confirmed in the diagnosis by allopaths, with but 3 deaths, a rate of but 1.4%, we can hardly understand a fixed minimum death-rate of 25%, much less a maximum rate of 95%, in a disease as readily amenable to the proper remedy as is pneumonia. The death-rate under the homoeopathic *similimum* should at no time exceed 5%, a higher rate would rather reflect on our ability.

It is with the hope of aiding the physician to find the *similimum* and to reduce his death-rate that this little *Monograph* is written.

The Authors.

320 Ontario Street,
Toledo, Ohio.

INTRODUCTION

This little *Monograph* has been divided into two parts—a Materia Medica and a Repertory.

The Materia Medica embraces the *leading* remedies that will be required in the greater majority of cases of pneumonia, covering all grades and types; it is divided into sections, as follows: The first section—REMARKS—aims to give a composite picture of the patient requiring that remedy and the remedy itself, together with other information regarding the remedy and the conditions requisite for its selection; the second section contains all the symptoms found under no other known remedy but the one under which they appear, and for which the remedy is given first rank, hence, they must be characteristic of the remedy under which they are found; the third section embraces all the symptoms for which the remedy is the only one given in the highest degree, hence the leader, and if there is no leader of the first degree, the ones in which the remedy is a leader are given.

The *graded* Repertory was added to supply whatever symptoms were for various reasons not admitted to the text, to use as a key to the text and to give at a glance the other remedies in the text having the same symptom and their relative values. In order to keep this Repertory within bounds it had to be confined strictly to the number of remedies in the text. The only remedies in the Repertory not graded are the ones under—Pneumonia and Pain. The remedies there given are of the first or highest grade only. All the remedies there listed were verified and graded by that Master Mind, the late, lamented James Tyler Kent, and are accurate and reliable.

Abbreviations and Signs: < = Agg., coming, increasing, worse, etc.; > = Amel., decreasing, better, going, etc.; a. = after; b. = before; d. = during; agg. = aggravation; amel. = amelioration; alt. = alternate, alternately, alternating, etc.; ext. = external, externally, extending; int. = internal, internally; l. = left; r. = right; esp. = especially. Remedies appearing in brackets in the Repertory, thus, [**Acon**], indicate that the remedy so appearing is of the highest grade and the only known remedy for that particular symptom. In all cases the shorter term will be used, thus: Sweat for perspiration, limbs for extremities, etc. This is all done to make the work as full as possible, to cut down the size for convenience in carrying compatible with accuracy, availability and reliability.

Remember that the SIMILIMUM will cut short any disease at any time and will act at once and rarely needs repetition. If it does need repetition it is NOT the *similimum*. The farther away you are from the similimum, the oftener you will have to repeat. Whenever a disease must run its, or a given, course it is a sign that you have at no time had the *simili-*

mum and that the patient would have been fully as well off, if not better, had he had no medical interference whatever.

We have tried to present each remedy in a manner which we believe will make the selection of the *similimum* a simpler and easier matter and fix the remedy more firmly in the mind of the prescriber.

DON'T: Get panicky; give too low potencies; repeat too often; paralyze your patient's heart with digitalis or ease his pains with morphine; try to replace the *similimum* with a tank of oxygen—they won't work.

MATERIA MEDICA

ACONITE (Acon.)

Remarks: Acon. automatically recalls a vigorous, plethoric, strong, robust individual, or a rugged, plethoric, rosy-cheeked child or infant whose troubles have come on suddenly and violently from violent exposure to cold, to cold air or to the dry, cold winds of midwinter, esp. the north, dry, cold winds, while thinly or insufficiently clothed and whose cases are characterized by extreme anxiety, restlessness, agonized tossing about, great fear, esp. of death; expression of anxiety and fear; extreme, unquenchable thirst for large quantities of water which agrees, everything else tastes bitter; expectoration rusty, or hot, bright blood or mucus heavily streaked with blood; cough comes suddenly; high fever; dry, hot skin; full, bounding, rapid pulse; sudden dyspnea with anguish; acute, sticking pains; must lie on back slightly elevated which >. "Agonized tossing about is essential to an Acon. case," T. F. Allen. Acon. affects the l. side, preferably the upper part. Its abuse calls for Bry. and esp. Sulf. After exudation starts Acon. is useless; it is then that such remedies as Bell., Bry., Iod., Sulf., etc., according to indications should follow.

Is the ONLY known remedy for: Pain cutting a. the chill; fever with one cheek red and hot, the other pale and cold; sense of boiling water poured into the chest.

Is THE leading remedy for: Thought he was about to die; fear in a crowd; nervous excitement; vertigo, swaying to r.; loud, barking cough; palpitation daytime, or a. fright; faintness a. urination; fever alt. with chill; sense of hot water in the chest.

ANTIMONIUM TART. (Ant-t.)

Remarks: Ant-t. automatically makes us think of children, old people, and esp. feeble people with broken down constitutions, always shivering, with pale, sickly faces; drawn, sunken noses; dark rings around the eyes; pale, shriveled lips; nostrils dilated, flapping, appear sooty inside; face cold, pale, covered with cold sweat, with a suffering expression; do not wish to be touched, looked at or talked to, esp. is this true of children; coarse rattling in chest, chest full of mucus but no or little expectoration, finally causing suffocation; drowsy; weak; cold sweat; pulse rapid, weak and trembling; coldness; relaxation; often must sit up in bed and be fanned (Carb-v., Tub); moan and whine piteously (esp. children); often sit up in bed, no clothing around neck or shoulders for both heat and bathing in cold water <; generally thirstless, do not like to have water offered; thick, ropy mucus is apt to fill up the mouth and choke the patient; dyspnea; threatening paralysis of lungs; cough usually short, without expectoration. Useful esp. in bilious, broncho, and one of the leaders in the pleuro and typhoid types. Follows Bry. and Ipec. well, coming in later, when the symptoms agree, esp. when the power of expulsion is almost gone. In the stage of great relaxation, coldness and prostration, cold sweat and little fever.

Is the ONLY known remedy for: Twitching in the face when coughing; profuse sweat on affected parts.

Is THE leading remedy for: Sleepiness with cough; abdominal respiration; asphyxia; dyspnea > expectoration.

ARSENICUM ALBUM (Ars.)

Remarks: When thinking of Ars. we naturally think of a weak, anemic, easily exhausted individual whose pneumonia is characterized by an anxiety with fear and restlessness almost equaling that of Acon., a restlessness that is more mental than physical, causing the patient to want to go from bed to bed; this restlessness soon changes into a profound prostration as in typhoid; rapid exhaustion, even collapse; burning, often as if coals of fire were in lung, or hot outside, cold inside (Reverse: Carb-v.); or surface of body usually cold, clammy and sweating; aspect and odors usually cadaverous; desires body kept warm and head cool; secretions usually acrid, odors putrid; desires to drink little and often; general < a. midnight, 1 a. m esp.; fears death (Acon.) and must have company;

the least exertion causes the most profound weakness; his expectoration is rusty or liver-colored. *Always study Sulf. in relation to Ars.*

Is the ONLY known remedy for: Anguish driving one from place to place; waking in fright at 3 a. m.; anxiety in stomach on rising up at night; twitching of lips when falling asleep; hiccough at the hour when the fever ought to come; oppression of the chest when the weather becomes cold or stormy; burning heat outside, coldness inside; sleeplessness from weariness; heat with chill absent 1 to 2 p. m., 12 to 2 a. m. or 1 to 2 a. m.; must sit up in bed with knees drawn up, resting head and arms on knees; stitching pains in apex of r. side; nausea 3 p. m.

Is THE leading remedy for: Anxiety at 3 a. m., or d. sleep, or d. sweat at night; despair d. sweat; attempt to escape, to change beds; fear of death when alone or of robbers; restlessness a. midnight, or d. chill, or wants to go from bed to bed; sadness when alone; unconscious from least motion, or in frequent spells; faint a. vomiting; pain in apex of r. lung; chill coming on at 1 to 2 a. m., or 12 to 2 p. m., or 1 to 2 p. m., or 2 p. m., or if drinking increases the chill with vomiting, or for the shaking chill in the night open air; fever, dry, coming on at night without thirst and with anxiety, or if it comes on at midnight or after, or at 12 to 3 a. m., or at 2 a. m., or 12 to 2 a. m., or 1 to 2 a. m.; irritative, slow fevers; sweat, night, with anxiety, or after the fever;

generally< 1 a. m.; weary a. eating; deep breathing impossible; dyspnea night in bed, or at midnight, or at 2 a. m., or on turning in bed; sleep restless a. 3 a. m.; sleepiness from mental exertion; thinks she is being watched; starting evenings on falling asleep; obstruction of nose at root, or with watery discharge; swelling of face morning; chilliness in pit of stomach; desire for warm food, and for warm drinks d. chill; nausea at 11 a. m., or a. fever; thirst for little and often; vomiting everything, or a. ice cream, or d. sweat; palpitation at 3 a. m., or irregular palpitation; drinking increases the chill and causes vomiting; sudden collapse, or collapse a. vomiting; burning, stitches internally.

BELLADONNA (Bell.)

Remarks: When one thinks of Bell. there comes to mind a vascular, plethoric, vigorous, intellectual individual or mentally active child whose complaints, like those of Acon., have come on suddenly and violently, stay any length of time and go as suddenly as they come, his pains and sweats esp. do so; burning heat and redness, to which dryness may be added, are very characteristic of Bell., the heat leaving a burning sensation to the examining hand; there is a high fever, always remittent, never continued; d. fever the bright red skin, usually shiny, becomes mottled as the fever advances; there is general throbbing, but esp. of the carotids; the pains are<

motion, jarring, light, noise and jar of bed; face is flushed; the pupils large, eyes glisten; great thirst, esp. for lemonade; generally < at 3 p. m.; takes cold from any draft of air; full, rapid pulse. Bell. prefers the r. side like Bry., but unlike Bry., Bell. cannot lie on the painful side. Infants laid on the painful side will turn to the opposite side immediately, a knowledge of which has helped us save several cases.

Is the ONLY known remedy for: Fear of animals; sits and breaks pins; burning heat alt. with chilliness, or int. and ext., body burning hot; sweat coming and going suddenly.

Is THE leading remedy for: Horrible visions; fear of imaginary things; desire to hide; kicking in sleep; laughing loudly, or sardonic; spitting in the faces of people; tearing things; distorted eyes, or convulsive movements; photophobia d. chill; pupils dilated d. heat; acute vision; red face while sitting; burning heat of face; risus sardonicus; tension in upper lip; desire for lemonade; cough from a sense of a foreign body in larynx, or racking night cough, or spasmodic cough afternoon; < lying on painful side; semi-conscious sleep; generally < 3 p. m.; > lying on abdomen; stitching pains transversely; from wetting head.

BRYONIA ALBA (Bry.)

Remarks: The Bry. subject, like the Acon. and Bell. subjects, is a plethoric individual whose complaints come on more slowly and go deeper. Before his troubles get started he complains of being tired, languid, does not wish to speak, be spoken to or move; the chill comes on a day or two after the exposure to cold; is more useful in the early stages and follows Acon. well, or if Acon. has been abused (Sulf); he is irritable, taciturn and is all business, esp. in typhoid states, talks and prattles about business, or thinks he is away from home and wants to go home, his delirium usually begins at 9 p. m. and lasts throughout the night (Bell. begins at 3 p. m. and lasts 'til midnight); face is generally besotted, purple, lips parched and dry; great thirst for large quantities, which if at long intervals makes Bry. the only known remedy; children desire things which they refuse when offered; grown people desire something, but know not what; high fever; profuse sweat; short, dry cough; rusty expectoration; generally > cool air and cool applications and esp. lying on affected side (Bell. reverse); is compelled to lie on r. side or back; the pains are sharp, stitching. Is one of the leaders in pleuro and typhoid types. Bry. has a marked affinity for the r. side and most complaints appear on that side.

Is the ONLY known remedy for: Unconscious morning on rising; thirst for large quantities of water at long intervals; chill beginning in lips; pain confined to the sternum.

Is THE leading remedy for: Talking of business; fear of poverty; desire to go home; quiet d. chill; sighing d. sweat; unconsciousness on rising up; chewing motion of jaw; vomiting > by drinking; thirst for large quantities and often; pain taking breath away; rough respiration; rheumatic pleurisy; > lying on painful side; pain in chest on sneezing, middle of chest > pressure of hand, in side d. cough, laughing or breathing; cutting pain in chest on inspiration or motion; pressing pain in chest d. cough; sore pain in chest > sitting upright, or under sternum on coughing; stitching pains in chest d. chill and fever > lying on affected side, or in sides > lying on affected side, or in lower part of sides < motion, or in sternum on coughing; r.-sided pneumonias; busy dreams or dreams of events of the previous day; chill beginning in finger tips; fever evening in bed, a. lying down, or at 9 p. m., or burning heat b. midnight, or with chill absent b. midnight; generally < 9 p. m.; > lying on painful side.

CALCAREA CARBONICA (Calc.)

Remarks: Calc. calls to mind fair, fat, flabby, sluggish individuals and children; or pale, anemic, waxy even though plump, with pale ears, lips and fingers pale and yellowish; anemic and chlorotic girls; chilly patients; cases esp. caused by working in water in which it follows Rhus well; patients who are sensitive to cold air and cold weather, esp. if damp;

his pains are < change of weather, esp. to damp; he is tired and < exertion of every kind; chilly, great relaxation; his thoughts keep him awake nights; cold sweaty hands and feet; face covered with cold sweat; children have a great longing for eggs; palpitation from every excitement; dyspnea from exertion; expectoration is sweetish and may be white or yellow and thick; ulcers on lungs; chest is very sore ext. to percussion or pressure, sharp pains shoot through it to back, it is also < inspiration; infants who sweat about the head and wet the pillow d. sleep and whose feet are cold and damp. Has a special affinity for and is the leading remedy for pneumonia of the r. upper lobe, and is adapted to the pleuro type.

Is the ONLY known remedy for: Delusion that people think her insane; inclined to grow fat (children); mind oversensitive when hearing of cruelties; desires boiled eggs; constriction and oppression of chest > drawing shoulders back; chill from working in clay.

Is THE leading remedy for: Delusions on closing eyes, or if frightful; exaltation of fancies nights; < when narrating her symptoms; photophobia evening; sneezing without coryza; dry cough before midnight; pneumonia r. upper lobe; chill beginning in scrobiculus cordis; chill from working in water; fever alt. with chill afternoon; weary of life d. sweat.

CARBO VEGETABILIS (Carb-v.)

Remarks: Carb-v. automatically calls to mind a lazy, sluggish, turgid individual with low vital powers, tending toward hemorrhage or putrid decomposition; in the collapsed stage when the patient wants to be fanned constantly with general fetid odors and bluish appearing skin; in the third stage with fetid expectoration, cold breath and sweat with desire to be fanned; veins lazy, relaxed and paralyzed; sluggish, lazy mind and body; excessive dyspnea with tendency to collapse; face purple, skin dusky; burning int., cold ext. (Reverse: Ars.); burning as from glowing coals; cold nose and knees; in spite of the fact that in collapse the face, breath and tongue are cold he must be fanned; his sleep is so full of anxiety that when he awakens he is covered with cold sweat; in last stages a peculiar death-like sleep with visions; face is pale, cold, lips pinched, nose pointed and drawn, or, face cold, pale and covered with sweat. Old, badly treated cases of pneumonia with a remaining bronchitis; where the hepatization has never been cleared up, bad places in lungs and bronchial tubes with weakness of chest < coughing. Threatened paralysis of lungs. The pains are accompanied by burning < coughing; oppression as of a load on chest. Desires cold water d. chill, but is thirstless d. fever. Where prolonged cold spells come on a. the fever has subsided somewhat and there is no reaction, vital powers low. In the language of the late

C. G. Raue: "Often at the brink of death, a savior."

The ONLY known remedy for: Weakness of chest on waking; ext. heat with desire to be fanned in place of thirst d. the heat; waking from cold limbs.

Is THE leading remedy for: Anxiety on closing eyes, or with heat of face; breathing impeded by flatulence; icy coldness of skin of whole body with cold breath; faintness on waking; distended stomach> eructations; weakness mornings on waking; dangerous cases where the whole body becomes icy cold, with cold breath; dyspnea> eructations, or with desire to be fanned, from flatulence.

CHELIDONIUM MAJUS (Chel.)

Remarks: Chel. calls to mind the bilious, lethargic, weak, weary individual who is indisposed to make any effort, with a sallow or yellowish-grey skin which gradually increases to jaundice; whites of eyes dirty yellow; yellow face< nose and cheeks; bitter taste; prefers hot food and hot drinks; slow pulse; aching pains involving the whole right lobe of the liver or the pain goes from the front of the liver or from the stomach to the back, but esp. to the lower angle of the r. scapula, which pains often become sharp, shooting; cases begin in r. side and ext. to l.; pleuro types with stitching, tearing pains; is as < from motion as Bry.; sits up in bed transfixed with pain, with high fever, bent forward on elbows holding himself perfectly still, < from both touch and motion; > heat, craves hot milk and fluids; chest > warm food; dyspnea; cough loose, rattling, expectoration difficult, grayish, scanty; fatiguing cough; short fits of coughing < change of weather. It selects the r. upper lobe (Calc.) and the l. lower lobe.

Is the ONLY known remedy for: Burning heat spreading from hands over whole body; general > noon a. eating and from hot milk.

Is THE leading remedy for: Red rash on chest; sore pain in r. side of chest; sweat 4 a. m. d. sleep.

FERRUM PHOSPHORICUM (Ferr-p.)

Remarks: Ferr-p. recalls an anemic, chlorotic, tired, weak individual, with much vascular excitement, who lacks vital heat and is sensitive to the open air, whose face is either red with congestion to the head d. fever or chlorotic, earthy, pale, sallow, pale lips, dark circles under the eyes. It vies with Acon. and Bell. for infants. It has been said that this remedy is a sort of cross between Acon. and Bell., as Cadmium between Ars. and Bry., and Seneg. between Bry. and Rhus. It is esp. useful in the congestive types with a vascular excitement simulating Verat-v. It has great oppression of chest; dyspnea; stitches in the chest on deep inspiration; short, spasmodic and very painful cough < lying; expectoration usually bloody; anxiety in and constriction of the chest and heart; chest < coughing and breathing, esp. deep breathing; the fever predominates; marked crepitus; it seems to have an affinity for the l. upper lobe. In the first stages of infantile pneumonia, esp. if caused by checked sweat on a summer day, also in adults before exudation; pulse full, round and soft; high fever; epistaxis and profuse expectoration of almost pure blood at the same time.

Is one of the leading remedies for: Earthy color of, or pale face; regurgitation of food; bloody expectoration; inflamed bronchial tubes; rapid pulse, and—*a more thorough proving.*

HEPAR (Hep.)

Remarks: Hep. automatically recalls a chilly subject who is extremely sensitive to ext. impressions and who is very, very hard to get along with; he is extremely sensitive to air, a draft, and, like Acon., to cold, dry winds; has profuse, easy sweating, the sweat usually of a sour odor, which does not > and in children the sour odor cannot be removed even by washing; he wants the clothing well drawn up about the neck, wants his sleeping room warm, is very quarrelsome, cannot endure the cold; if he gets cold at night in bed his complaints come on or are <, even the exposure of a hand or foot < ; he is full of sharp pains of a splinter-like, jagging character; his cough is generally

<evening until midnight with gagging, choking and sweat, but like Ant-t. there is often difficulty in removing the expectoration though the cough sounds loose and rattling. After exposure to cold or cold, dry winds the Hep. patient comes down more slowly than does the Acon. patient, therefore, Hep. follows Acon. well in such cases when the symptoms agree. Abscess of the lungs when the symptoms agree, .also, chronic cases of pneumonia with profuse, purulent expectoration and threatening abscess. Adapted well to the pleuro type.

Is the ONLY known remedy for: Closing the eyes nights excites cough; hoarse cough evening until midnight; cough in west wind.

Is THE leading remedy for: Disposition to contradict; weeping d. cough; heat of the face evening and night; desire for vinegar; hacking cough a. dinner; suffocative cough night; cough in the wind, cold, dry, east or north; chill 6 p. m. until 5 a. m.; sweat day and night without>; sour sweat night or profuse sweat day and night without>.

IODUM (Iod.)

Remarks: Iod. suggests a scrofulus, warm-blooded individual who is anxious both bodily and mentally, the last coming on esp. if he tries to keep still; excitement; sense of heat, desires to be bathed in cold water or have face cool sponged. Iod. must be carefully differentiated from Acon. and Bry., it lacks the extreme anxiety of Acon. and comes in later d. the stage of hepatization and it lacks the sticking pains of Bry., but has the high fever of both; the cough is dry; affects the apex by preference; suffocates in a warm room d. the hot stage; dreads the heat; if able to be up and around is hurried and would like to walk continually; sweats easily and is easily exhausted; desires room cool. Pericarditis complicating pneumonia. Is generally hungry and < if he fasts. Pleuro types.

Is the ONLY known remedy for: Ravenous appetite 3 hours a. eating; double quartan chill with diarrhea on days free from fever.

Is THE leading remedy for: Eructations daytime; heavy food <.

IPECACUANHA (Ipec.)

Remarks: Ipec. makes us think of infants and children for whose pneumonia it is the leading remedy; little ones who look pale and dreadfully sick, blue rings around the eyes; anxious; nose drawn; dangerous dyspnea; the coarse rattling can be heard all over the room; cough dry, racking, teasing, suffocative, causing redness of face, gagging, choking and inclination to vomit without nausea; thirstless; there may be occipital pains d. chill; restless, tosses about; prostration comes in spells. Cases often ushered in or accompanied by nausea and vomiting. Cases coming on earlier than Ant-t. and not having the coldness of Ant-t., corresponding to the stage of irritation, while Ant-t. corresponds to the stage of relaxation.

Is the ONLY known remedy for: Stiffness of muscles of face d. cough; suffocative cough at 7 p. m.; pressing pain in diaphragm; short chill, long heat, no thirst.

Is THE leading remedy for: Vomiting a. stooping; child becomes stiff and blue in the face with suffocative cough; pneumonia of infants; chill from disordered stomach.

LOBELIA INFLATA (Lob.)

Remarks: Lob. usually calls to mind a light complexioned, fleshy, dyspeptic individual with relaxed muscles, whose case is characterized by deathly nausea, faint, weak stomach; oppression of heart and chest; cough with sneezing, gaping and flatulent eructations; spasmodic contraction of diaphragm; as if heart would stand still; pulse frequent but small; as of a band about chest; dyspnea extreme, < slightest exertion; urine generally deep red, depositing a copious, red sediment; cases esp. associated with heart troubles or intermittents. Intermittent forms, esp. in individuals who live in malarial districts, accompanied by affections of broncho or heart, dyspnea with apprehension of death, with strong constriction of middle of chest, or from least exertion; nausea with cold sweat on face or profuse flow of clammy saliva; spasmodic contraction of diaphragm. Broncho cases. Infants. Neglected cases.

Is the ONLY known remedy for: Emptiness and sinking at stomach ext. to heart.

Is THE leading remedy for: Breathing difficult in or from cold air; sensation as if the heart would cease to beat.

Is one of the leaders for: Pale face; deathly nausea; paroxysmal vomiting; breathing asthmatic, spasmodic, difficult while lying; expectoration of mucus; affections of the heart; constriction of the chest; chill at noon; emaciation of old people, and—*a more thorough proving.*

LYCOPODIUM (Lyc.)

Remarks: Lyc. brings to mind old, tired people with feeble reaction who are sensitive to cold, < cold, cold air, cold food, cold drinks, from exertion and 4 to 8 p. m.; whose faces are sallow, sickly, pale, often withered, shriveled and emaciated and whose foreheads wrinkle with every pain, jar or noise, whose nostrils flap, but are not as wide open nor sooty inside like Ant-t.; dyspnea < exertion; flatulence; faintness; rattling of mucus in chest or dry, hacking cough without expectoration; easy satiety or eating < the appetite: chest filled with mucus; inability to expectorate; inability to lie on back. Double pneumonia beginning on r. side, ext. to 1. Neglected cases with dyspnea from accumulation of serum in pleura and pericardium. In hepatization it closely resembles Phos. and Sulf. (see Sulf). Esp. useful for old people with feeble reaction and weakness of all functions and who do not tend to convalesce, and children who are extremely cross on waking. After the pneumonia the dry cough remains a long time or there is much asthmatic and whistling respiration, cold limbs, head and face hot, wants to go with head uncovered. Elects the r. side or goes from r. to l. and is one of the leaders for neglected and typhoid cases. Very valuable for children who look wrinkled and prematurely old.

Is the ONLY known remedy for: Weeping 4 to 8 p. m., or when thanked; obstruction of nose with pus nights; face wrinkled with chest symptoms; anxiety in stomach a. vexation; eating increases the appetite and the hunger, also d. aversion to food; dry cough in emaciated boys, chronic in pining boys; cough overpowering, as if the larynx were tickled by a feather evening b. sleep.; burning heat 4 p. m. lasting several hours;> in general a. midnight; pain in sides of chest at 4 p. m.

Is THE leading remedy for: Anger evening; dulness of mind> open air; irritability morning on waking; laughing d. sleep; restlessness in room, and while sitting; weeping aloud; fan-like motion of alae nasi in pneumonia; obstruction of nose d. sleep; confused expression on face; bitter eructations a. eating, food comes up; nausea from fasting; thirst a. sweat; breathing arrested nights, or difficult while lying on back; cough evening on going to sleep; palpitation d. digestion; shocks in chest with cough; waking from hunger; chill 4 to 8 p. m.; fever 6 to 8 p. m.;> in general forenoon;< eating onions; pulse frequent a. eating;< in general 4 p. m. and esp. 4 to 8 p. m.; loathing of life mornings.

MERCURIUS (Merc.)

Remarks: Merc. naturally calls to mind a weak, trembling, restless, apprehensive individual who talks hurriedly and who is extremely sensitive to the extremes of either heat or cold and < from the heat of the bed and esp. at night, who is always sweating and is< thereby, who is< lying on the r. side, has fetid breath, offensive saliva, offensive sweat having a rather sweetish, penetrating odor, his cough is< lying on the r. side, skin is sallow and he recovers slowly, cough usually at night and is loose. Infantile lobar cases. It elects esp. the r. lower lobe. Useful in bilious and broncho forms. The expectoration is bloodstreaked; tongue yellow, soon becoming dry.

Is the ONLY known remedy for: Photophobia from light of fire; emptiness of and sinking at stomach from pressure; sweat, daytime with nausea and languor, or cold sweat with anxiety while eating, or warm sweat becoming cold and sticky a. stool.

Is THE leading remedy for: Restlessness 8 p. m.; photophobia from gaslight; epistaxis d. sleep; heat of face with chilliness; swelling of cheeks; black tongue, edges red; pale tongue; desires bread and butter; stitches in anterior part of chest, also on coughing; chill as of water poured over one; fever paroxysmal nights; sweat nights oily; < lying on r. side; gnawing pains.

NATRUM SULFURICUM (Nat-s.)

Remarks: Nat-s. calls to mind a bilious, sickly-looking individual with a sycotic or hydrogenoid constitution who cannot stand any dampness as it either brings on or < all his symptoms; esp. useful if he lives near a waterway, and is usually, if not always, accompanied by liver complications < lying on the l. side (Merc., the r.), he is sensitive to touch, pressure, the night air and to pain, his pains are > motion, and he is usually at his worst d. rest, in the spring and in warm weather, the skin is jaundiced, the mouth always slimy, his dyspnea and oppression of the chest always < dampness and > open air, the cough usually < 3 or 4 a. m., and the chest is > holding it with both hands, the expectoration is glairy, the tongue usually has a dirty, grayish-green coat at the root, or brown if jaundice complicates. It selects esp. the l. lower lobe.

Is the ONLY known remedy for: Loathing of life, must restrain herself from doing herself bodily injury; redness of eyelids at night; greenish-gray tongue; sycotic pneumonia.

Is THE leading remedy for: Cheerful a. stool; photophobia d. headache; green tongue; dyspnea of children, or in wet weather; oppression of heart while sitting; pain in chest in damp weather; < green vegetables.

PHOSPHORUS (Phos.)

Remarks: Thinking of Phos. automatically recalls to mind a feeble subject, mentally and physically exhausted, with trembling of limbs and subject to vertigo, who, born sick, grows up rapidly and slender; delicate, waxy, anemic, emaciated subjects with earthy, sunken, pale, haggard, anemic faces; chlorotic girls; patients who are vehement, irascible; who are < in general from cold, cold applications, sweets, in cool, damp or hot weather, from wetting feet and esp. hands, and > warmth and warm applications except the head and stomach; and who are sensitive to all ext. impressions, and desire to be rubbed, are always tired, are > a. sleep, have fanlike motion of alae nasi, great thirst for ice-cold drinks, desire cold food which > the stomach; have anxiety, constriction, oppression, weakness of, and sensation of a load lying on the chest; chest > lying on the r. side, violent stitching pains in l. chest, the expectoration of bright red blood, bloodstreaked, rusty or purulent, in later stages thick, yellow, sweetish. Cases characterized by great oppression of chest, heaviness as from a load, burning in chest and head, hot cheeks, fever, gesticulations and delirium, violent thirst for cold drinks, fan-like motion of alae nasi, dyspnea, catchy respiration, lies on back with head thrown far back, short, dry cough and constriction of chest. Bronchial catarrh a. pneumonia. Hepatization with dry, hacking cough; Kent says, "Sulf., Lyc., and Phos. are the most frequently indicated remedies for the hepatization d. pneumonia; Phos. follows Ars., when the symptoms agree, or when Ars. was suited to the restlessness, prostration and anxiety but can do no more on account of the hepatization"; then comes in Phos. for the thirst for ice-cold water, constriction of the chest, dry, hacking cough, paralytic weakness of the lungs and expectoration of bloody, frothy mucus. Kent reports a typical Phos. pneumonia, as follows: "Burning in chest and head, hot cheeks and fever; gesticulation and delirium; violent thirst for ice-cold water; fan-like motion of alae nasi; dyspnea; respiration catchy; short, dry cough; rawness in chest, bruised feeling; pains cutting, burning or sharp and tearing in lungs d. cough; suffocation or almost impossible inspiration, esp. at the beginning of hepatization, when face becomes livid, features pointed, cold sweat and quick, hard pulse." Expectoration frothy in low typhoid forms. Threatened paralysis of lungs. Is indicated after febrile symptoms have mostly subsided, when there is great oppression of chest as from a weight, esp. if < lying on the l. side. Elects esp. the r. lower lobe. Is useful for infants and neglected cases and one of the leaders for the: Broncho, pleuro and typhoid types.

Is the ONLY known remedy for: Epistaxis with sweat; nausea from putting hands in warm water; anxiety in chest from excitement; constriction of sternum when coughing; hepatization of lung > lying on r. side, < lying on l.; pain in lower chest lying on l. side, stitching in l. side > lying on r. side; chest becoming immovable; breathing becoming stridulous evening on falling asleep.

Is THE leading remedy for: Anxiety while lying on the l. side, or d. a thunderstorm; fear d. a thunderstorm; motion slow; sympathetic; persistent epistaxis; dryness of center of tongue; appetite increased d. fever; desires ice cream; emptiness at stomach d. nausea; eructations paroxysmal, of food by the mouthful; vomiting as soon as water becomes warm in stomach; cough dry, < lying on l. side or reading aloud, or tickling cough in open air, or tight, or coughing on going from cold to warm air or vice-versa; constriction of chest d. cough; pain in chest on rising up in bed, > warmth, in sides lying on l. side, in lungs, l., lower, rawness in cold air; palpitation evenings, on rising from bed or a seat; sleep lying on r. side, impossible on l.; burning heat with thirst for cold drinks; salt<; superficial respiration.

PULSATILLA (Puls.)

Remarks: Puls. automatically calls to mind the plethoric, mild, tearful, gentle, yielding, changeable, fidgety individual who is easily irritated, touchy and always feeling slighted, who is< in a warm or crowded room and in the evening, who craves the cool open air and if able to move about must move slowly, who is thirstless, who must wear the thinnest of clothing even in moderately cool weather (which is similar to its antidote—Sulf.), whose face is sickly, often intermixed with yellow and of an unhealthy color; chlorotic individuals, chilly, burning heat at night without thirst, palpitation, longing for fresh air and other Puls. symptoms; there is general <evenings, beginning to move and from lying on the l. and painless side,> from slow motion, cold places, lying on the painful side (Bry.) and from cold drinks. Catarrhal pneumonias. Cases complicated with suppressed menses. Anxiety evening and night, while lying on l. side; fullness about heart; fever 2 p. m. followed by chill at 4 p. m.; burning heat intolerable at night in bed; distended veins and burning hands that seek cool places; sweat comes on d. the stupid sleep at night; thirstless; dyspnea; dry, teasing cough at night;

wants windows and doors wide open, must have fresh air; palpitation while lying on l. side.

Is the ONLY known remedy for: Anxiety as if in hot air; transiently unconscious afternoon in a warm room; cotton-like mucus in mouth; nauseous taste after smoking; meat tastes putrid; eructations tasting of bad meat or rancid tallow; thirst at 2 p. m.; cough exhausting, nights, disturbing sleep; anxiety in chest while lying on l. side; fullness of heart evening; fever at 2 p. m. followed by chill at 4 p. m. or at 2 p. m. with chill absent, or dry heat with distended veins and burning hands that seek cool places; sweat lasting all night with loquacity, or night d. stupid sleep; distended blood vessels evening; pain in part recently lain on; stretching b. urination; weakness morning while lying; cases complicated with suppressed menses.

Is THE leading remedy for: Delirium with sleepiness; fear in evening twilight; moaning d. the heat; sadness in warm room; oversensitive d. heat; unconscious in warm or crowded room; weeping > open air; obstruction of nose evening; sneezing in warm room; sweat of face d. heat; dryness of tongue without thirst; offensive odor of mouth mornings; saliva cotton-like; bitter taste evening, or d. eating, or a. swallowing food, or a. smoking, or clammy taste or clay-like, or nauseous morning; sticky after-taste; eructation evening and night, bitter at night, of fluid, or nauseous; nausea a. ice cream, or with suppressed menses, or a. pork; dyspnea with suppressed menses; loud breathing in sleep; cough constant evenings, cough on exertion, or exhausting cough nights, or cough when becoming heated; expectoration morning on rising, tasting of an old catarrh or nauseous; anxiety in chest evening and night; oppression of chest> open air, of heart evening; pain in chest> bending forward, on lying on sound side, in lower chest, in heart evening, pressing in heart evening, sore below clavicle, wandering stitches; palpitation a. supper; sleep lying on abdomen, overpowering sleepiness afternoons; sleeplessness evening from heat or from activity of thoughts, same idea always repeated; yawning b. menses; chill afternoon following heat, or evening a. lying down or with the pains, or b. midnight; chilliness evening; chill< warm things; fever afternoon a. lying down, 2 p. m. or evening on entering the warm room; sweat morning a. heat;< in general evening twilight; faintness in a close or crowded room;< bread and butter; weakness morning in bed, or on waking, or in warm room.

RHUS TOXICODENDRON (Rhus)

Remarks: Rhus naturally recalls the rheumatic individual whose troubles have been brought on from exposure to cold, damp weather and to cold, damp air while perspiring, such as ice-handlers or workers in water, who are< from rest, on beginning to move, on rising from a seat and from cold, are> from warmth and motion but easily fatigued from continued motion (Puls. differs that it must move slowly to avoid the heat which<), > change of position, he is extremely restless because he cannot find a comfortable place in bed and therefore must move to ease his pains, there is general soreness, stiffness and lameness. There is a general tendency to become typhoid. Cases marked by stitching pains, intense fever, marked thirst, great prostration, dyspnea and bloody expectoration. Useful in both pleuro and typhoid forms.

Is the ONLY known remedy for: Dwells on past disagreeable occurrences a. midnight; triangular red tip of tongue, or white on one side, or yellow white at base; dreams of roaming over fields; fever 10 a. m. as if dashed with hot water, or hot water running through bloodvessels.

Is THE leading remedy for: Timid and irritable at night; eyes closed; tongue brown morning; desire milk; dyspnea 6 p. m.; cough< bathing, or b. chill, dry; restless sleep a. midnight; chill from becoming wet, when overheated; heat of l. side, r. cold; < in general cloudy weather; weakness sitting; cases from getting wet, esp. d. sweat; breath hot; weeping without knowing why.

SANGUINARIA (Sang.)

Remarks: Sang. calls to mind phthisical subjects who have a previous history of migraine and who have been much debilitated by chronic bronchial catarrh, who have been subject to taking cold with every change of the weather, esp. to damp, or from a change of clothing; patients with burning palms and soles like Sulf., circumscribed red spots over the malar bones and burning cheeks, who come down suddenly with a chill, dry, harsh, violent cough, every cough felt as a concussion at the bifurcation of trachea, as if a knife were in the part or as if torn asunder, every cough ending in belching, great dyspnea, cough < lying down, cough > discharging flatus up and down, patient particularly > lying on the back, burning in the chest, rusty expectoration. Adapted esp. to the subacute types, and esp. to hypostatic pneumonias (Verat-v.). In the typhoid types the face becomes livid and dark red. It selects either side.

Is the ONLY known remedy for: Dry cough > discharge of flatus up and down and with this must sit up. Cough in general > eructations and passing of flatus.

Is THE leading remedy for: Cough from crawling in throat-pit; cough from dryness in larynx, or hacking cough afternoons; pain behind sternum.

SENEGA (Seneg.)

Remarks: The Seneg. individual is of necessity of the catarrhal type whose being dwells intimately around the respiratory organs and whose sufferings are sharp and acute from taking cold, in cold weather esp. In its pleuropneumonias it comes in in cases too deep for Bry. As Ferr-p. is sort of a cross between Acon. and Bell., and as Cadm. is sort of a cross between Ars. and Bry., so is Seneg. a sort of cross between Bry. and Rhus. The violent symptoms simulate those of Bry. but there is >motion,< rest. The chest pains are> motion, but the cough is <motion. The rattling in the chest is as marked as that of Ant-t. and Ipec., but not so loud as Ipec. The expectoration is as copious, gluey and sticky as Kali-bi., and as hard to raise as Caust., so that it must be swallowed. Chest pains< d. rest and when inspiring and when lying on r. side. Cough usually< evening and night, in warm room and lying on r. side. Expectoration of tough mucus. Soreness of chest walls< coughing, pressure, sneezing or moving arms; stitches and rattling of mucus in chest; dyspnea; congestion of lungs, etc. Profuse secretion of lungs in old people even with no other symptoms. Pleuro cases with exhaustion as extreme as that of Ars. and Phos. Esp. useful for old people.

Is the ONLY known remedy for: Pain behind sternum when walking fast; clawing pain in chest.

Is THE leading remedy for: Pain in chest while sitting.

SEPIA (Sep.)

Remarks: Sep. recalls the anemic, chlorotic individual, esp. with dark hair, or the tall, slim woman with a narrow pelvis, who is excitable, nervous, fidgety, who brooks no opposition, whose appearance is anemic, waxy, sallow, skin mottled with yellow or freckled face, face flabby, who is < company yet dreads being alone, who is stupid, dull, thinks slowly, constipated, cannot sleep on the l. side because of palpitation, who is generally < forenoon and evening, from washing in water and at rest; oppression of chest and weak, empty, sinking feeling at stomach. This characteristic emptiness with nausea as soon as she thinks of food, the yellow saddle across the nose and upper part of cheeks, a distressing feeling as of a lump in the rectum make the choice of Sep. an assured fact.

Is the ONLY known remedy for: Yellow saddle across cheeks; emptiness at stomach evening > a. eating, also when thinking of food; constant cough night on waking; pain sticking in short ribs; faintness with heat then coldness; weakness > d. menses.

Is THE leading remedy for: Aversion to husband, members of family and to business; > when alone, averse to company; > when occupied; cracked lower lip; saddle across nose;

emptiness at stomach d. headache; nausea b. breakfast; constant cough, night, lying down; violent cough evening a. lying; oppression of chest morning; chill without subsequent heat or thirst; cold sweat night; faintness d. chill, or on exertion, or d. fever; general heat afternoon and evening.

SILICA (Sil.)

Remarks: Sil. calls to mind, like Hep., a chilly individual whose face is anemic, sickly, tired, waxy, lips rough, cracked and peeling, like Puls., he is mild, yielding, tearful, but irritable when aroused and the children cross when spoken to, there is general < at night, from open air, cold and wet, lying on painful side, wine, pressure and change of weather, > from warmth and wrapping up and usually in cold, dry weather, the cough is increased by ice cream, cold water and cold things in general to gagging and dreadful retching; flushes of heat and rattling in chest. It follows Puls. well and is deeper acting. It is mostly called for in the suppurative stage with muco-purulent expectoration, also old people with offensive expectoration. Don't overlook the offensive feet. Is a leader in neglected cases.

Is the ONLY known remedy for: Catching respiration night and d. fever; cough on uncovering feet.

Is THE leading remedy for: Obstruction of the nose with pus; thirst at night; catching respiration; dreams of previous and long past events; sleeplessness from orgasms of blood; chilliness lasting all day; <in general from feet becoming cold.

SULPHUR (Sulf.)

Remarks: Sulf. recalls vividly the light complexioned people esp., as well as those who have very red lips as well as redness of other orifices of body, often with soreness and burning; scrofulous individuals; those who have harsh, rough skins, coarse hair, are weak and liable to eruptions; who have disagreeable odors emanating from the body with general < from and aversion to bathing; chilly individuals who have no reaction in hepatization, want to lie still; individuals who are angular, dyspeptic, hungry, lank, lean and stoop-shouldered, or even if fat, rotund and well fed; of sedentary habits; or if dirty, shriveled, red faced, always red and dirty looking, children never look as if washed clean; uncleanly, careless about their attire; annoyed by offensive odors yet do offensive things, the odors of their own bodies annoy them; their lungs burn, the tops of their heads burn, their soles burn at night so that they must put their feet out of bed, their urine burns on passing; they are < at night and from the warmth of the bed; are faint and hungry around 11 a. m., eat little and drink much; flushes of heat rise from chest to head. Useful after Brv. if the patient does not rally and the symptoms agree. Valuable in the later stages when the inflammatory processes fail to resolve, the lung continues dull, the cough dry, the patient begins to have fever at night, feet, hands and head hot. Kent says, "If all at once at 1-2 or 3 a. m. the patient begins to sink, his nose becomes pinched, his lips drawn, he takes on a hippocratic countenance, is covered with cold sweat, is too feeble in every part of his body to move and only moves his head a little in a restless manner, unless you give him a dose of Ars. at once he will die, this will warm him up and make him feel that he is going to get well, but as soon as this is accomplished you must give him at once the antidote which is Sulf., or you will fail; or if after Ars. the patient rallying goes into a fever, hot fever coming on with a burning thirst and he cannot get enough ice-cold water then follow with Phos." If after the attack there is a lingering cough and the patient has never felt well since his pneumonia and is chilly Sulf. will clear up his case. Sulf. is always to be thought of when the supposedly well chosen, but unfortunately only apparently indicated, remedy has acted only partially and then either fails to hold or to go on and finish up the case (or Tub. if Sulf. fails or the symptoms are continuously changing). If it has any special affinity whatever it is for the l. lower lobe. Follows Acon. well and is its leading antidote, esp. for its abuse. Of the very highest value in neglected cases, a leader in typhoid cases and quite important in pleuro cases.

Is the ONLY known remedy for: Anxiety from pressure on chest; indifference to welfare of others; smell acute to stool; heat of face with shivering; nausea at odors of his own body; respiration difficult and oppression of chest on bending arms backward; flushes of heat in chest rising to face; pain burning in chest ext. to face; pulsation in chest night on waking.

Is THE leading remedy for: Anxiety night on waking; indifference to ext. things; restless b. menses; odors b. nose offensive, of snuff; smell acute to unpleasant odors; sneezing evenings; red lips; hunger increased 11 a. m., or with weakness, or vanishes at sight of food; appetite wanting with thirst; desires raw food; emptiness at stomach b. dinner; respiration difficult evening; cough dry nights, $<$ lying, loose by day, also on waking, or cough b. sleep, or disturbing sleep; expectoration of mucus morning; fullness of chest b. menses; itching in axilla; pain burning in chest ext. upward, or sticking, sticking ext. to back, or from clavicle to scapula, or from sides to scapula, or in l. side on inspiring and ext. to back or scapula, or in sides ext. to scapula, or in heart ext. to scapula; palpitation $<$ motion of arms, or on going to sleep, or on turning in bed; sense of warmth in chest; weakness of chest from loud talking; nightmare when lying on back; dreams unpleasant; sleeplessness a. 5 a. m.; unrefreshing sleep morning; waking from dreams, or frequent waking a. midnight; chill predominating at noon; sour sweat morning; profuse sweat morning a. waking and with sleeplessness; < in general 11 a. m.; faintness 11 a. m.; weakness afternoon.

TUBERCULINUM (Tub.)

Remarks: Tub. naturally brings to mind the tubercular, feeble patient who is anemic, pale, nervous, waxy, always tired, whose symptoms are kaleidoscopic, ever-changing; when our deepest acting remedies act but a short time and must be changed, one who has inherited tuberculosis, whose case either relapses or changes symptoms. The cases are characterized by bruised soreness all over, even eyeballs, subject to cold sweat on head, face becomes red, even purple, d. chill, thirst d. chill and heat for large quantities of cold water, all gone, faint, hungry feeling at stomach, aversion to meat, desire for milk, dry, hacking cough b. chill, desire for fresh air, < warm room, cold, cold damp weather or becoming cold, > motion (esp. if Rhus fails), mentally restless. It follows Calc. and Rhus well. Like Rhus it has a dry, hacking cough that preceeds the chill and comes in after Rhus, if Rhus fails to permanently > the cough. It is a deeper acting remedy than Sulf., and like Sulf. to be thought of when the supposedly well chosen, but unfortunately only apparently indicated remedy, has acted only partially and then either fails to hold or to go on and clear up the case, even after Sulf. has failed in this condition. [Diphtherinum, Tuberculinum and Variolinum: They remove the predisposition to diphtheria, tuberculosis and smallpox respectively as no other known remedies or methods can do and in a manner that is not only effective but an unmixed blessing to humanity. The removal of the predisposition to any disease is the only true and safe method of disease prevention. The futile attempt to prevent disease by the present crude methods now in force can never be otherwise than disastrous and the ever increasing death-rate from heart failure attests and confirms our statement.]

Is THE leading remedy for: Red face afternoons; weakness from nightsweats.

Is ONE of the leading remedies for: Dulness of mind; epistaxis; face red, circumscribed, or pale, sickly color; heat of face; desires delicacies and smoked meats; thirst d. heat; cough dry or hacking; expectoration thick, yellow; oppression of chest; chilliness with sweat or from putting hands out of bed, shivers if he uncovers, aversion to uncovering; hectic fever; heat with sweat, chilly if uncovering; sweat a. midnight, also if profuse; < in general bathing, change of weather, cold to warm; tendency to take cold; emaciation; general heat with sweat; weariness; > in general warm bed.

VERATRUM VIRIDE (Verat-v.)

Remarks: Verat-v. recalls at first glance a patient that might be mistaken for a Bell. subject, who has great arterial excitement, dilated pupils, flushed, livid face, dry mouth, tongue and lips, the characteristic red streak down the center of the tongue, full, hard, quick, strong pulse, throbbing headache, dyspnea, breathing labored and slow, cerebral congestion, heart beat loud and strong and often a sinking, faint feeling at pit of stomach, lungs engorged, cough, expectoration usually bloody or clear, bloody mucus, high fever, threatened cardiac paralysis from overexertion of heart, generally indicated, like Acon., before hepatization has taken place when it will quite frequently abort the whole trouble.

Is THE leading remedy for: Vomiting a. cold water.

Is ONE of the leading remedies for: Delirium; face bluish, or red; vomiting; coldness in general; cold sweat; rapid pulse, also irregular, and slow.

THERAPEUTIC HINTS

Each remedy seems to have its own characteristic stamp:

Acon.: The agonized tossing about.

Ant-t.: The aversion to being looked at, touched or spoken to.

Ars.: The thirst for little and often.

Bell.: The burning heat and redness.

Bry.: The great thirst for large quantities at long intervals.

Calc.: The cold, sweaty feet and hands.

Carb-v.: The desire to be fanned.

Chel.: The constant pain under the lower angle of the r. scapula.

Ferr-p.: The anemic face easily flushed. Intercurrent pneumonias (Boger).

Hep.: The prolonged sour sweat without >.

Lob.: The great oppression around the heart with gastric symptoms.

Lyc.: The 4 to 8 p. m. <.

Merc.: The nightly < with inability to lie on r. side.

Phos.: The thirst for ice-cold water.

Puls: The thirstlessness.

Rhus: The triangular, red tip of the tongue.

Sang.: The 2 to 4 p. m. fever.

Seneg.: The mixed symptoms of Bry., Kali-bi. and Rhus.

Sep.: The yellow saddle across the nose ext. to cheeks.

Sil.: The offensive sweat, esp. of axillae and feet.

Sulf.: The constant heat on top of head with burning soles and red orifices.

Tub.: The ever-changing symptoms.

Verat-v.: The red streak down the center of the tongue.

Note: A remedy not mentioned in this work, but to be thought of in cases where the patient is dull, stupid, has little reaction and complains of no pain or discomfort is **Opium.** Dr. Boger claims this remedy to be of great value in such cases which he calls "do nothing" cases.

Another remedy not mentioned, but which is to be thought of in cases on a septic base is Pyrogenium when there are symptoms which appear to be a mixture of Arn., Eup., and Rhus and where the temperature and pulse do not correspond, the pulse being rapid, irregular and fluttering.

REPERTORY

PNEUMONIA: Acon, Ant-t, Ars, *Bell,* **Bry,** *Calc,* **Carb-v, Chel, Ferr-p, Hep,** *Iod, Ipec,* **Lob, Lyc, Merc,** *Nat-s,* **Phos, Puls, Rhus,** *Sang,* **Seneg, Sep,** *Sil,* **Sulf,** Tub, **Verat-v. Right:** *Bell,* **Bry,** *Chel, Lyc, Merc, Phos, Sang;* lower lobe: *Merc, Phos;* upper lobe: **Calc,** *Chel.* **Left:** *Acon, Calc, Nat-s,* Phos, *Sang,* Sulf; lower lobe: *Chel, Nat-s,* Sulf; upper lobe: *Acon.* **Aconite,** abuse of, after: *Bry,* Sulf. **Aged** persons: *Bry, Nat-s, Seneg.* **Infants:** *Acon, Ant-t, Bry, Ferr-p,* **Ipec,** *Lob, Lyc, Merc, Phos.* **Lie** on back, must: Acon Sulf. **Lying** on back, with head thrown back: Phos; lying on back>: Acon, Phos, Sulf. **Menses** suppressed [**Puls**]. **Neglected:** *Lob,* **Lyc,** *Phos, Sang, Sep,* **Sil, Sulf. Pleura: Ant-t, Bry,** *Calc, Hep, Iod,* **Phos,** *Rhus, Seneg, Sulf.* **Sycotic:** [**Nat-s**]. **Typhoid: Ant-t, Bry, Lyc, Phos,** *Rhus, Sang,* **Sulf.**

MIND

Anger: Acon, Ars, *Bell,* **Bry,** *Calc, Carb-v,* Chel, Ferr-p **Hep,** *Iod, Ipec,* **Lyc,** Merc, *Nat-s, Phos,* Puls, *Rhus,* Sang, Seneg, **Sep,** Sil, **Sulf.**

Anguish: Acon, Ant-t, **Ars, Bell, Calc,** *Carb-v,* **Hep,** *Phos,* Puls, Sep; driving from place to place: [**Ars**].

Answers: Irrelevantly: Bell, Carb-v, **Phos, Sulf; refuses:** Ars, Bell, **Phos, Sulf; slowly:** Ars, *Carb-v,* **Merc, Phos,** *Rhus,* Sep, *Sulf.*

Anxiety: Acon, *Ant-t,* **Ars, Bell, Bry, Calc, Carb-v,** *Chel,* Ferr-p, *Hep,* **Iod,** Ipec, **Lyc,** *Merc,* **Phos, Puls, Rhus,** Sang, *Seneg, Sep, Sil,* **Sulf; morning: Ars,** *Carb-v,* Ipec, *Lyc,* **Phos,** Puls, Rhus, Sep, *Sulf;* **evening:** Acon, Ant-t, **Ars,** Bell, Bry, **Calc, Carb-v,** Chel, *Hep, Lyc, Merc, Phos, Puls, Rhus,* **Sep,** Sil, **Sulf,** in **bed: Ars,** *Bry, Calc,* **Carb-v,** Hep, *Lyc,* Phos, *Puls,* Sep, Sil, *Sulf;* **night:** *Acon,* **Ars,** *Bell,* Bry, *Calc, Carb-v,* Ferr-p, *Hep,* Lyc, *Merc, Phos,* **Puls,** *Rhus,* Sep, Sil, *Sulf,* on **waking:** *Ars,* Carb-v, Chel, Lyc, *Phos, Puls,* Sil, **Sulf; midnight, a.: Ars,** Calc,

Hep, Lyc, *Rhus*, **3 a. m.: Ars,** Sil; **alone,** when: **Ars, Phos; bed,** in: **Ars,** *Bry*, *Calc*, *Carb-v*, *Hep*, *Lyc*, Phos, *Puls*, **Rhus,** Sep, Sil, *Sulf*; **chill,** d.: **Acon, Ars, Calc,** Carb-v, Phos, **Puls,** *Rhus*, Sep; **fear,** with: **Acon,** Ant-t, **Ars,** Bell, Bry, *Calc*, Chel, Ferr-p, *Hep*, *Lyc*, *Merc*, *Phos*, *Puls*, *Rhus*, *Sep*, Sulf; **fever,** d.: **Acon, Ars,** Bell, *Bry*, *Calc*, Ferr-p, Hep, **Ipec,** Merc, *Phos*, *Puls*, *Rhus*, **Sep,** Sulf; **house,** in: Ars, *Bry*, Chel, **Lyc, Puls, Rhus; lying** on l. side: **Phos,** Puls; **menses, d.:** Acon, *Bell*, Calc, Merc, Phos, **Sil,** Sulf; **noise,** from: Chel, Puls, **Sil; pressure** on chest: **[Sulf]; sleep,** d.: Acon, **Ars,** *Bell*, Hep, *Lyc*, Merc, *Phos*, Puls, Rhus; **thunderstorm,** d.: **Phos,** Sep; **waking,** on.: Acon, **Ars,** Bell, Calc, *Carb-v*, Hep, Ipec, Lyc, *Phos*, Puls, Rhus, Sep, Sil, *Sulf*.

Business: Talks of: Ars, Bell, **Bry,** Phos, Sulf.

Company: Aversion to: > alone: Ferr-p, *Lyc*, Phos, **Sep,** Sulf; **desires: Ars,** Bell, Bry, *Calc*, Carb-v, Hep, **Lyc,** Merc, **Phos,** *Puls*, *Sep*, < while alone: **Ars,** Calc, *Lyc*, **Phos,** Sil.

Confusion of mind: *Acon*, *Ant-t*, *Ars*, **Bell, Bry, Calc, Carb-v,** *Chel*, Ferr-p, Hep, Iod, Ipec, Lob, *Lyc*, **Merc,** Nat-s, *Phos*, *Puls*, **Rhus,** Sang, *Seneg*, **Sep, Sil,** *Sulf*; **morning:** Acon, Ant-t, Ars, Bell, *Bry*, *Calc*, *Carb-v*, Chel, Ferr-p, Iod, Lyc, Merc, Nat-s, Phos, *Rhus*, Seneg, Sep, Sil, **Sulf;** compelled to **arouse** himself: **Carb-v,** Sulf; **eating,** a.: Bell, *Calc*, *Carb-v*, Ferr-p, Lob, *Lyc*, *Merc*, *Phos*, **Puls,** *Sep*, *Sil*, *Sulf*; **waking,** on: Acon, Ant-t, Ars, Bry, Calc, *Carb-v*, Chel, Hep, *Lyc*, Merc, **Phos,** *Puls*, Rhus, *Sep*, *Sil*, *Sulf*; **warm** room, in: Acon, Bell, *Iod*, **Lyc,** Phos, **Puls,** *Sulf*.

Consolation: <: *Ars*, *Bell*, Calc, Lyc, Merc, **Sep, Sil.**

Contradiction: Disposed to: **Hep,** *Lyc*, Merc; **intolerable:** Acon, Ars, *Bry*, **Lyc,** Merc, **Sep,** *Sil*.

Death: Presentiment of: **Acon,** Ars, *Bell*, Bry, Calc, *Chel*, *Hep*, *Lyc*, Merc, *Phos*, Puls, Rhus, Sep; **thoughts** of: **Acon,** *Ars*, Chel.

Delirium: *Acon*, Ant-t, **Ars, Bell, Bry,** *Calc*, Carb-v, **Chel,** Hep, Iod, *Ipec*, Lob, **Lyc,** *Merc*, *Phos*. *Puls*,

Rhus, Sil, *Sulf,* **Verat-v; daybreak: Bry; night: Acon, Ars,** *Bell, Bry,* Calc, Carb-v, *Chel,* Hep, Lyc, *Merc, Puls,* Sep, Sil, Sulf; **frightful:** *Acon,* **Bell,** Calc, *Phos, Puls,* Sil; **muttering:** Ars, *Bell,* **Bry,** Chel, *Hep, Lyc, Merc,* **Phos,** *Rhus;* **quiet: Bry,** *Carb-v, Chel,* Phos, Rhus; **sleep,** d.: Acon, Ars, **Bell,** Merc; **sleepiness,** with: Acon, *Bry,* **Puls; violent:** *Acon,* **Ars, Bell,** Phos, Puls; **wild: Bell.**

Delusions: *Acon, Ars,* **Bell,** Bry, *Calc,* Carb-v, Iod, *Lyc, Merc, Phos, Puls, Rhus,* Sep, *Sil,* **Sulf; die,** that he was about to: **Acon,** *Chel,* Rhus; **faces,** sees: Ars, **Bell,** *Calc,* Carb-v, Merc, Phos, *Sulf,* on closing eyes: Ars, **Bell,** *Bry,* **Calc,** Carb-v, Sulf.

Despair: *Acon,* Ant-t, **Ars,** Bell, Bry, **Calc,** Carb-v, Chel, Hep, Iod, *Lyc, Merc,* Nat-s, *Puls, Rhus,* Sep, Sil, *Sulf;* **chill,** d.: *Acon,* Ant-t, **Ars,** Bell, Bry, *Calc,* Hep, Merc, Rhus, *Sep;* **sweat,** d.: **Ars,** Calc, *Carb-v,* Lyc, *Sep;* **recovery,** of: *Acon,* **Ars,** *Bry,* **Calc,** *Sep,* Sil.

Discontent, displeased, dissatisfied: Acon, *Ars,* Bell, *Bry,* Calc, *Chel,* Ferr-p, *Hep,* Iod, Ipec, *Lyc,* **Merc,** Phos, *Puls, Rhus, Sep, Sil,* **Sulf.**

Dwells on past disagreeable occurrences a. midnight: [**Rhus**].

Escape, attempts to: Acon, *Ars,* **Bell,** *Bry,* Merc, Phos, Puls, Rhus, Sulf, Tub.

Excitement: Acon, Ant-t, *Ars,* **Bell,** *Bry, Calc,* Carb-v, *Chel, Ferr-p, Iod, Lyc, Merc,* **Phos, Puls,** Rhus, Sang, Seneg, *Sep, Sil, Sulf,* Tub; **chill,** d.: **Acon,** Ars, Calc, Carb-v, *Hep,* Lyc, Phos, Puls, Sulf; **nervous: Acon,** Phos.

Fear: Acon, Ant-t, *Ars,* **Bell,** *Bry,* **Calc,** *Carb-v,* Ferr-p, *Hep, Iod,* Ipec, Lob, **Lyc,** *Merc,* **Phos,** *Puls, Rhus,* **Sep,** Sil, *Sulf;* **evening:** Ant-t, *Ars,* **Calc,** *Carb-v,* Hep, *Lyc,* Merc, *Phos,* **Puls,** *Rhus,* **twilight:** *Calc, Phos,* **Puls,** Rhus; **night:** *Ars, Bell, Calc, Carb-v,* Hep, Ipec, Lyc, *Merc,* Phos, *Puls,* **Rhus,** Sil, *Sulf;* **alone,** of being: Ant-t, **Ars,** Bell, Bry, Calc,

Hep, **Lyc,** Merc, **Phos,** *Puls*, *Sep*; **death,** of: **Acon,** Ant-t, **Ars,** *Bell*, *Bry*, **Calc,** *Ferr-p*, *Hep*, Ipec, Lob, *Lyc*, **Phos,** *Puls*, *Rhus*, Sep, Sulf, Verat-v, when alone: **Ars,** Bell, *Phos*; **people,** of: *Acon*, Ars, Bell, Calc, *Carb-v*, Ferr-p, Hep, *Iod*, **Lyc,** Merc, Phos, *Puls*, **Rhus,** Sep, Sulf; **poverty,** of: **Bry,** *Calc*, Puls, *Sep*, Sulf; **robbers,** of: **Ars,** Bell, *Merc*, *Phos*, Sil, Sulf.

Frightened easily: *Acon*, Ant-t, **Ars,** *Bell*, *Bry*, *Calc*, *Carb-v*, **Lyc,** *Merc*, *Phos*, *Puls*, Rhus, **Sep,** *Sil*, *Sulf*; **wakens** at 3 a. m.: [**Ars**].

Home, desires to go: Bell, **Bry,** *Calc*, Rhus.

Impatience: *Acon*, *Ars*. Bell, *Bry*, *Calc*, Carb-v, *Hep*, *Iod*, *Ipec*, *Lyc*, Merc, *Puls*, *Rhus*, Sang, **Sep,** *Sil*, **Sulf.**

Indifference: *Acon*, Ant-t, *Ars*, *Bell*, *Calc*, **Carb-v,** *Chel*, Ferr-p, Hep, Iod, Ipec, *Lyc*, *Merc*, **Phos, Puls,** Rhus, Seneg, **Sep,** *Sil*, *Sulf*; **chill,** d.: **Phos,** Puls, Sil; **everything,** to: *Acon*, Bell, **Carb-v,** *Merc*, *Phos*, *Sep*, Sulf; **ext.** things, to: Lyc, **Sulf.**

Irritability: **Acon,** *Ant-t*, *Ars*, **Bell, Bry, Calc, Carb-v,** Chel, Ferr-p, **Hep,** *Iod*, *Ipec*, **Lyc,** *Merc*, *Nat-s*, **Phos, Puls, Rhus,** Sang, Seneg, **Sep, Sil, Sulf,** *Tub*, **Verat-v;** **morning** on waking: Ars, *Bell*, Bry, **Lyc,** *Puls*, Rhus, *Sulf*; **evening:** Ant-t, *Calc*, *Lyc*, Phos, *Puls*, Sil, **Sulf;** **night:** Lyc, Phos, **Rhus;** **chill,** d.: Acon, *Ars*, Bell, Bry, **Calc,** Carb-v, Hep, **Lyc,** Merc, Phos, *Puls*, *Rhus*, Sep, Sil, *Sulf*; **<consolation:** *Bell*, Calc, Lyc, Merc, **Sep, Sil.**

Lamenting, bemoaning, bewailing, etc.: *Acon*, *Ars*, *Bell*, *Bry*, *Calc*, Ipec, **Lyc,** Merc, Phos, *Puls*, Rhus, Sep, Sil, *Sulf*, **Verat-v.**

Laughing: Loudly: **Bell;** **sleep,** d.: **Lyc,** Sep, *Sil*, Sulf.

Loathing of life: Ant-t, **Ars,** *Bell*, *Calc*, *Carb-v*, Hep, *Lyc*, **Merc,** *Nat-s*, **Phos,** *Puls*, *Rhus*, *Sep*, *Sil*. *Sulf*.

Mildness: *Acon*, **Ars,** Bell, *Calc*, Chel, Iod, *Lyc*, *Phos*, **Puls, Rhus,** *Sep*, **Sil,** *Sulf*.

Moaning, groaning, etc.: **Acon,** Ant-t, *Ars*, **Bell,** *Bry*, Calc, Carb-v, *Ipec*, Merc, *Phos*, *Puls*, Rhus, Sulf.

Morose: Bell, **Bry,** *Calc*, Carb-v, Chel, Ferr-p, *Ipec*, *Lyc*, *Merc*, *Phos*, **Puls,** Sang, **Sil,** *Sulf*.

Prostration of mind: Ars, *Bry*, *Calc*, *Carb-v*, *Hep*, Iod, **Lyc,** Merc, **Phos,** *Puls*, Rhus, Seneg, **Sep, Sil, Sulf,**

Quiet, desires to be: Bell, **Bry; chill,** d.: Ars. **Bry.**

Restlessness, nervous: **Acon,** *Ant-t*, **Ars, Bell.** Bry, **Calc,** *Carb-v*, *Chel*, Ferr-p, *Iod*, *Ipec*, Lob, **Lyc, Merc,** Nat-s, Phos, **Puls, Rhus, Sep, Sil, Sulf; 8 p. m.:** Calc, **Merc; night:** Acon, Ant-t, **Ars,** *Bell*, Bry, *Calc*, *Carb-v*, Ferr-p, Iod, **Lyc, Merc,** Nat-s, *Phos*, **Puls, Rhus,** Sang, *Sep*, Sil, **Sulf,** Verat-v; **midnight,** a.: **Ars,** Lyc, Sil, Sulf; **anxious:** *Acon*, **Ars,** *Bell*, *Bry*, *Calc*, *Carb-v*, Chel, *Hep*, Iod, *Merc*, *Phos*, *Puls*, *Rhus*, Sep, *Sil*, *Sulf*; **bed,** drives one out of: **Ars,** *Bell*, Bry, Ferr-p, *Hep*, *Lyc*, Merc, Puls, **Rhus,** Sep, Sil, wants to go from bed to bed: **Ars,** *Bell*, *Calc*, Merc, *Rhus*, Sep, tosses about in bed: *Acon*, Ant-t, **Ars,** *Bell*, *Bry*, *Calc*, Ferr-p, *Lyc*, *Merc*, Phos, *Puls*, **Rhus,** *Sep*, *Sulf*; **chill,** d.: Acon, **Ars,** *Bell*, Carb-v, Rhus; **heat,** d.: *Acon*, Ant-t, **Ars,** *Bell*, Calc, *Carb-v*, Ferr-p, *Ipec*, *Lyc*, **Puls, Rhus,** *Sulf*; **int.:** Acon, **Ars,** Chel, Lob, Lyc, Phos, **Rhus,** Sep, **Sil; menses,** b.: Acon, Lyc, Puls, **Sulf; room,** in: *Iod*, **Lyc.**

Sadness: Acon, Ars, *Bell*, *Bry*, **Calc,** *Carb-v*, *Chel*, *Ferr-p*, *Hep*, **Iod,** *Ipec*, Lob, **Lyc, Merc, Nat-s,** *Phos*, **Puls, Rhus,** Sang, Seneg, **Sep,** *Sil*, **Sulf,** *Verat-v*; **evening:** Ant-t, *Ars*, *Calc*, *Carb-v*, Ferr-p, *Hep*, *Lyc*, *Phos*, **Puls,** Rhus, Seneg, *Sep*, *Sulf*; **alone,** when; **Ars,** *Calc*, Lyc, Phos, Sil; **chill,** d.: **Acon. Ars,** Calc, Hep, *Lyc*, Merc, Phos, *Puls*, Rhus, Sep; **heat,** d.: **Acon, Ars,** *Bell*, Bry, *Calc*, Lyc, Nat-s, *Phos*, Puls, *Rhus*, Sep, *Sil*, Sulf; **menses,** b.: Bell, *Calc*, Ferr-p, *Lyc*, Phos, **Puls,** *Sep*; **warm** room: Calc, **Puls,** Rhus.

Senses acute: **Ars, Bell, Phos.**

Sensitive: *Acon*, *Ars*, **Bell,** Bry, *Calc*, *Carb-v*, Ferr-p, Hep, *Iod*, **Lyc,** *Merc*, *Nat-s*, **Phos, Puls,** *Seneg*, *Sep*, **Sil, Sulf; noise,** to: **Acon.** Ant-t, *Ars*, **Bell,** *Bry*,

Calc, *Carb-v*, Chel, *Ferr-p*, Iod, *Ipec*, *Lyc*, *Merc*, *Nat-s*, *Phos*, *Puls*, Rhus, **Sep, Sil.**

Shrieking: Acon, Ars, *Bell*, Bry, *Calc*, Carb-v, *Ipec*, **Lyc,** Merc, *Phos*, Puls, Seneg, Sep, Sil, *Sulf*, *Tub*; **pain,** with the: **Acon,** *Ars*, **Bell,** Puls; **sleep,** d.: Bell, *Bry*, Calc, Chel, Hep, Ipec, **Lyc,** Phos, **Puls,** Sep, Sil, *Sulf*; **urination,** b.: **Lyc.**

Sighing: Acon, Bell, *Bry*, *Ipec*, Puls, *Rhus*, Sulf; **sweat,** d.: Acon, Ars, **Bry,** *Ipec*, Phos, *Rhus*, *Sep*.

Speech: Hasty: Acon, Ars, *Bell*, Bry, **Hep,** Lyc, **Merc,** *Sep*; **incoherent:** Ars, *Bell*, **Bry,** Chel, Hep, Merc, **Phos, Rhus,** *Sulf*; **prattling: Bry; unintelligible:** Acon, Ars, **Bell,** Lyc, *Merc*, Sil; **wandering:** Acon, *Ars*, **Bell,** *Bry*, Calc, **Lyc,** Merc, *Phos*, *Puls*, *Rhus*, *Sulf*.

Starting: *Acon*, Ant-t, **Ars, Bell, Bry,** *Calc*, *Carb-v*, Chel, Hep, *Lyc*, Merc, *Phos*, Rhus, *Sep*, *Sil*, *Sulf*; **evening** on falling asleep: **Ars,** *Bell*, Bry, *Sulf*; **fright,** from: *Acon*, **Bell,** Bry, *Carb-v*, *Lyc*, *Merc*, **Nat-s,** *Phos*, *Sep*, *Sil*, *Sulf*; **noise,** from: Ars, *Calc*, Carb-v, Chel, *Lyc*, *Merc*, **Nat-s,** Rhus, **Sil,** Sulf; **sleep,** on falling to: **Ars, Bell,** Bry, Carb-v, **Hep,** Ipec, **Lyc,** Merc, *Nat-s*, *Phos*, Sep, *Sil*, **Sulf,** Tub; **sleep,** from: *Acon*, Ant-t, *Ars*, **Bell,** Bry, Carb-v, Chel, *Hep*, Lyc, *Merc*, *Phos*, *Puls*, Sang, *Sep*, *Sil*, *Sulf*.

Stupefaction: Acon, Ant-t, *Ars*, **Bell, Bry,** *Calc*, Chel, Ferr-p, Iod, Ipec, *Lyc*, Nat-s, **Phos,** *Puls*, **Rhus,** Seneg, Sep, Sil, *Sulf*.

Talk: Indisposed to: *Acon*, *Ars*, *Bell*, Bry, *Calc*, *Carb-v*, Chel, Ferr-p, *Hep*, Iod, Ipec, *Lyc*, Merc, *Nat-s*, **Phos, Puls,** *Rhus*, Sep, Sil, **Sulf;** of others <: **Ars,** *Nat-s*, Rhus, *Sep*, Sil.

Unconscious: **Acon,** Ant-t, *Ars*, **Bell,** *Bry*, Calc, *Carb-v*, *Chel*, *Hep*, Ipec, *Lyc*, Merc, *Phos*, **Puls,** *Rhus*, Sep, *Sil*, *Sulf*, Verat-v; **morning: Bry,** Chel, Lyc, Phos, Sulf, on rising: [**Bry.**]; in crowded **room:** Ars, *Lyc*, *Phos*, **Puls,** Sulf; **frequent** spells: **Ars,** *Phos*; least **motion: Ars, rising** up: **Bry,** *Carb-v*, **transient:** Calc, Chel, Hep, **Puls,** Sil, afternoon in warm room: [**Puls**]; **warm** room: *Acon*, *Lyc*, **Puls.**

Weary of life: **Ars,** *Bell,* Calc, Carb-v, Hep, Lyc, Merc, **Phos,** *Puls, Rhus,* Sep, *Sil,* Sulf; **sweat,** d.: **Calc,** Hep, *Merc,* Sil.

Weeping: *Acon, Ant-t,* Ars, *Bell, Bry,* **Calc,** *Carb-v,* Chel, Ferr-p, *Hep, Iod,* Ipec, Lob, **Lyc,** Merc, *Nat-s, Phos,* **Puls, Rhus, Sep,** Sil, **Sulf; 11 a. m.:** [**Sulf**]; **4 to 8 p. m.:** [**Lyc**]; **aloud: Lyc,** Phos, Puls, Sulf; alt. with **laughter:** *Acon,* Bell, *Calc, Lyc,* **Merc,** *Phos, Puls,* Sep, Sulf; **causeless:** Ars, Bell, *Lyc,* **Puls, Sulf,** without knowing why: **Rhus,** Sep; **chill,** d.: Acon, Ars, **Bell, Calc,** *Carb-v,* Hep, **Lyc,** Merc, **Puls,** Sil, Sulf; **<consolation:** Bell, Calc, Lyc, Merc, **Sep, Sil,** Sulf; **cough,** b.: Ant-t, **Bell, Bry, Hep, d.:** Ant-t, Ars, *Bell,* **Hep,** Ipec, Lyc, Sep, Sil, Sulf; **heat,** d.: **Acon, Bell,** Bry, Calc, Ipec, *Lyc,* **Puls,** Sulf; **involuntary:** *Bell,* Merc, Phos, **Puls, Rhus, Sep; sweat,** d.: Acon, **Bell,** Bry, *Calc,* **Lyc,** Phos, *Puls,* Rhus, Sep, Sulf.

EYES

Brilliant: *Ars,* **Bell,** *Lyc,* Puls.

Distorted: *Acon, Ars,* **Bell,** Carb-v, *Chel, Merc,* Puls, *Sil, Sulf,* Verat-v.

Dull: Acon, **Ant-t,** Ars, Bell, Bry, Calc, *Carb-v.* Iod, *Lyc, Merc,* Phos, Rhus, Sang, *Sulf.*

Open lids: Ant-t, **Iod, Lyc; half:** *Ant-t, Ars,* **Bell,** *Bry,* Ferr-p, *Ipec, Lyc, Merc, Phos, Rhus, Sulf.*

Photophobia: Acon, *Ant-t,* **Ars, Bell,** *Bry,* **Calc,** *Chel, Hep,* Ipec, **Lyc, Merc, Nat-s,** *Phos, Puls,* **Rhus,** Seneg, *Sep, Sil,* **Sulf,** *Tub;* **evening: Calc,** *Lyc, Merc,* Sil; **chill,** d.: Acon, Ars, **Bell,** Hep, Lyc, Rhus, Sep; **daylight:** *Acon,* **Ars,** Bell, *Bry, Hep, Lyc, Merc, Phos,* Sep, Sil, *Sulf;* light of **fire:** [**Merc.**], of **sun: Acon,** *Ars, Bry,* Calc, *Hep, Merc, Phos,* **Sulf.**

Pupils dilated: *Acon,* Ars, **Bell, Calc,** *Chel,* Hep, *Iod,* Ipec, Lyc, *Merc, Phos, Puls, Sang,* Sulf.

Staring: *Acon, Ant-t, Ars,* **Bell,** Bry, *Calc,* Carb-v, *Hep,* **Iod,** Ipec, **Lyc, Merc,** Phos, Puls, Rhus, Sang, Seneg, Sil, Sulf.

Sunken: Ant-t, *Ars,* Bell, Calc, *Carb-v,* Chel, Ferr-p, Iod, *Lyc, Merc, Phos,* **Puls,** Sang, Sep, *Sulf.*

Swollen: *Acon, Ars, Bry,* Carb-v, *Hep, Ipec,* Lyc, Merc, Phos, Puls, **Rhus, Sep; morning:** Bry, **Sep,** Sil, **Sulf.**

NOSE

Dilated nostrils: *Ant-t, Ars, Lyc,* Phos.

Motion of wings fan-like: *Ant-t, Chel, Iod,* **Lyc,** *Phos, Sulf.*

Smell acute to strong odors: *Acon,* **Bell,** Bry, Calc, *Hep,* **Lyc, Phos,** Puls, *Sep, Sulf,* to **flowers:** Lyc, **Phos,** Sang, to **food: Ars,** *Ipec,* **Sep.**

Sneezing: *Acon, Ant-t,* **Ars,** *Bell,* **Bry,** *Calc,* **Carb-v,** Chel, *Ferr-p,* Hep, *Iod, Ipec, Lyc,* **Merc,** *Nat-s, Phos,* **Puls, Rhus, Sang,** *Seneg, Sep, Sil,* **Sulf; morning:** Bry, Calc, Lyc, Merc, Phos, *Puls, Sep,* **Sulf; evening:** *Iod,* Phos, *Puls,* **Sulf; frequent:** Acon, **Ars,** *Bell, Bry,* Calc, **Carb-v,** *Hep, Lyc,* **Merc,** *Phos,* Rhus, *Sang,* Sep, *Sil,* **Sulf; ineffectual:** Acon, Calc, **Carb-v,** Lyc, Phos, **Sil,** Sulf; **uncovering,** from: **Hep,** *Merc, Rhus,* hands: **Hep,** Rhus; **warm** room: **Puls.**

Sooty nostrils: *Ant-t, Lyc.*

FACE

Chlorotic: Ars, *Bell,* **Calc,** *Carb-v,* Ferr-p, **Lyc,** Merc, *Phos,* **Puls, Sep, Sulf.**

Congested: Acon, Ant-t, **Bell,** *Bry, Calc, Iod, Phos,* **Puls.**

Discoloration: Ashy: *Ars, Phos,* Sulf; **black** lips: Acon, Ant-t, **Ars,** Bry, *Carb-v, Merc, Phos,* Rhus; **bluish** d. chill: Bry, Sulf, *Tub,* d. cough: Bell, **Ipec,** lips d. chill: *Ars, Ipec;* **changing** color: *Acon,*

Ars, Bell, **Phos,** Puls; **cynaotic: Ars, earthy:** *Ant-t, Ars,* Bell, *Bry, Calc, Carb-v,* **Ferr-p,** Iod, Ipec, *Lyc,* **Merc,** *Phos, Puls,* **Sep,** *Sil,* Sulf; **grayish:** *Ars, Carb-v, Chel,* **Lyc,** Phos, yellow: *Carb-v,* Chel. **Lyc; greenish:** *Ars,* **Carb-v, Chel,** *Iod,* Merc, *Puls;* **pale:** *Acon,* **Ant-t, Ars,** *Bell, Bry,* **Calc, Carb-v,** *Chel,* **Ferr-p,** *Iod, Ipec,* **Lob, Lyc,** *Merc,* Nat-s, *Phos, Puls, Rhus, Sang,* **Sep,** *Sil,* **Sulf, Tub,** Verat-v, d. **chill:** Bell, **Bry,** *Hep,* Ipec, *Lyc,* Phos, *Puls, Rhus,* Sep, *Sulf,* d. **heat:** *Ars, Ipec, Lyc,* Puls, Rhus, Sep, lips: Ant-t, **Ars,** *Calc, Ferr-p,* Ipec, *Lyc, Puls,* Sulf, Verat-v; **red: Acon,** *Ant-t, Ars,* **Bell, Bry,** Calc, Carb-v, **Chel,** *Ferr-p, Hep,* Iod, Ipec, Lob, *Lyc, Merc,* Nat-s, **Phos,** *Puls,* **Rhus, Sang,** *Sep, Sil, Sulf,* **Verat-v,** afternoon: Sang, **Tub,** circumscribed: Acon, *Ant-t, Ars,* Bry, Calc, Carb-v, Chel. Ferr-p, Hep, Iod, **Lyc,** Merc, **Phos,** *Puls, Sang,* Seneg, Sep, Sil, **Sulf, Tub,** d. cough: Acon, **Bell,** Bry, *Carb-v,* Hep, *Ipec,* Lyc, **Sang,** Sil, Sulf, d. fever: **Bell,** Chel, Ferr-p, Ipec, Lyc, Merc, Phos, Rhus, Sang, **Sep,** Sil, Sulf, *Tub;* **sallow:** *Ars, Calc,* **Carb-v, Chel,** Ferr-p, *Iod, Merc, Nat-s,* Puls, *Sep,* **Sulf; sickly** color: **Ars, Calc,** *Carb-v, Chel, Iod,* **Lyc,** *Merc,* Nat-s, *Phos,* Rhus, Sil, *Sulf,* **Tub; yellow:** Acon, **Ars,** *Bell, Bry,* **Calc,** *Carb-v,* **Chel,** *Ferr-p, Hep, Iod, Ipec,* **Lyc, Merc. Nat-s,** *Phos, Puls,* Rhus, **Sep,** *Sil,* **Sulf.**

Drawn: *Acon,* **Ars, Bell,** *Bry,* Calc, *Carb-v,* Chel, Hep, Iod, *Ipec,* **Lyc,** *Merc, Phos,* Puls, *Rhus,* Sep, Sil, *Sulf.*

Expression: Anxious: **Acon,** *Ant-t,* **Ars,** *Bell, Calc, Carb-v, Chel, Lyc,* Merc, *Sulf;* **confused:** *Ars,* **Lyc,** Phos; **distressed: Ars,** *Iod,* Phos; **fear: Acon,** Ars; **haggard: Ars,** Bell, *Carb-v,* Merc, *Phos,* Sang, *Sil, Verat-v;* **sickly:** Acon, **Ars,** *Calc, Carb-v, Chel, Iod,* **Lyc,** *Merc,* Nat-s, *Phos, Rhus,* Sep, *Sil, Sulf, Tub;* **suffering:** *Acon, Ant-t,* **Ars,** *Carb-v, Chel, Phos, Puls,* **Sil, Sulf.**

Heat: *Acon, Ant-t,* Ars, **Bell, Bry,** *Calc, Chel, Ferr-p,* **Hep,** *Ipec, Lyc, Merc, Phos,* **Puls,** *Rhus, Sang,* Seneg, *Sil, Sulf,* **Tub; evening:** *Acon,* Ant-t, Bry, **Hep,** Lob, Lyc, Phos, Puls, Rhus. Sep, Sil, *Sulf;*

night: Hep; anxiety, d.: **Carb-v; burning:** Acon, **Bell,** *Bry*, Chel, Iod, Rhus, *Sang*, Sulf; **chilliness,** d.: **Merc; flushes:** *Acon*, Ars, *Chel*, Ferr-p, Hep, Lob, **Lyc,** *Phos*, Rhus, Seneg, **Sep,** *Sil*, **Sulf,** with shivering: [**Sulf**].

Hippocratic: Acon, **Ant-t, Ars, Carb-v,** Ferr-p, Iod, Lyc, Merc, *Phos*.

Sweat: Acon, Ant-t, *Ars*, **Bell,** *Bry*, **Calc, Carb-v,** Ferr-p, Hep, *Ipec*, **Lyc, Merc,** *Nat-s*, *Phos*, **Puls,** Rhus, *Sep*, **Sil,** *Sulf*, Verat-v; **cold:** Acon, *Ant-t*, **Ars,** Bell, *Bry*, *Calc*, **Carb-v,** Hep, *Ipec*, *Lob*, *Lyc*, *Merc*, *Puls*, Rhus, Sep, *Sulf*, Verat-v; **heat,** d.: *Chel*, **Puls; one-sided: Puls,** Sulf.

Picking lips: **Bry.**

Sordes on lips: **Ars,** *Phos*.

Sunken: Acon, **Ant-t, Ars,** Bell, *Calc*, **Carb-v,** *Chel*, Ferr-p, Iod, *Ipec*, *Lyc*, *Merc*, *Nat-s*, *Phos*, *Rhus*, Sep, *Sulf*.

Swollen: Morning: **Ars,** Calc, Merc.

Twitching: Coughing, when: [**Ant-t**]; upper **lip:** *Ars*, **Carb-v,** of lips on falling asleep: [**Ars**].

Wrinkled with chest symptoms: [**Lyc**].

STOMACH

Appetite: Capricious: Ars, Bell, **Bry,** *Hep*, *Ipec*, *Phos*, *Puls*, *Sang*, *Tub*; easy **satiety:** Ant-t, Ars, Bry, **Lyc,** Merc, *Phos*, Rhus, *Sep*, *Sil*, *Sulf*; **increased:** 11 a. m.: *Iod*, **Sulf,** night: Bry, **Lyc, Phos,** Puls, Sulf, d. chill: **Ars,** *Phos*, **Sil,** a. eating: Acon, *Calc*, **Lyc,** *Merc*, **Phos,** eating< the: [**Lyc**], d. fever: **Phos,** vanishing at sight of food: *Phos*, **Sulf,** with weakness: Merc, *Phos*, **Sulf; insatiable: Iod, Lyc,** *Sep*; **ravenous:** 11 a. m.: *Iod*, **Sulf,** night: Bry, *Lyc*, **Phos,** Sep, Sil, Sulf, soon a. eating: Acon, *Calc*, **Iod, Lyc,** *Merc*, **Phos,** *Sulf*; without **relish** until he begins to eat: **Lyc; wanting** at sight of food: *Phos*, **Sulf,** with thirst: Ant-t, Ars, *Calc*, *Phos*, Rhus, Seneg, Sep, Sil, **Sulf.**

Aversion to: Butter: Ars, Carb-v, *Merc*, *Phos*, **Puls,** Sang; warm **drinks: Phos, Puls;** fat and rich **food:** *Ars*, Bell, *Bry*, Calc, *Carb-v*, *Hep*, *Merc*, Phos, **Puls,** Rhus, Sang, *Sep*, *Sulf*; **smell** of food: *Ars*, **Ipec,** *Sep*; to **food** until he tastes it and then he is ravenous: [**Lyc**]; **warm** food: *Bell*, *Calc*, *Lyc*, Merc, **Phos, Puls,** *Sil*; **meat:** *Ars*, Bell, *Bry*, **Calc,** *Carb-v*, Chel, Ferr-p, *Lyc*, *Merc*, Nat-s, *Phos*, **Puls,** *Rhus*, **Sep, Sil, Sulf,** *Tub*.

Desires: Alcoholic drinks: Acon, Ant-t, **Ars,** Bry, Calc, *Hep*, *Iod*, *Lyc*, Merc, *Phos*, *Puls*, *Sep*, **Sulf,** *Tub*; **beer: Acon,** Ars, *Bell*, *Bry*, Calc, Chel, *Merc*, *Nat-s*, Phos, *Puls*, *Rhus*, Sep, **Sulf; whiskey:** Acon, *Ars*, Calc, Hep, Merc, *Phos*, Puls, **Sulf; wine:** *Acon*, *Ars*, *Bry*, *Calc*, Chel, *Hep*, Merc, **Phos,** Puls, *Sep*, **Sulf; bread** and butter: Bell, **Merc,** Puls; cold **drinks: Acon,** *Ant-t*, **Ars,** *Bell*, **Bry,** *Calc*, Chel, *Lyc*, **Merc, Nat-s, Phos,** Puls, *Rhus*, *Sep*, Sulf; **delicacies:** Calc, **Ipec,** *Rhus*, Sang, **Tub;** highly **seasoned** food: *Hep*, **Phos,** Puls, *Sang*, Sep, **Sulf; ice cream:** *Calc*, **Phos,** Tub; **indistinct,** knows not what: **Bry,** Ipec, **Puls,** Sang, Sil; **lemonade: Bell,** Calc, Puls; smoked **meat: Tub; milk:** *Ars*, *Bry*, *Calc*, *Chel*, *Merc*, **Rhus,** *Sil*, Sulf; **raw** food: Sil, **Sulf; salt** things: *Calc*, **Carb-v, Phos,** Sulf, Tub; **sour** things: *Ant-t*, *Ars*, Bell, *Bry*, *Calc*, *Carb-v*, Chel, Ferr-p, **Hep,** *Phos*, *Puls*, Rhus, *Sep*, *Sulf*; **sweets:** Ars, *Bry*, *Calc*, *Carb-v*, *Ipec*, **Lyc,** Merc, *Rhus*, *Sep*, **Sulf,** *Tub*; **vinegar:** Ars, Chel, **Hep,** *Sep*, Sulf; **warm** drinks: **Ars,** Bell, **Bry,** Carb-v, *Chel*, *Lyc*, *Sulf*, d. chill: **Ars,** food: **Ars,** *Chel*, *Lyc*, Sil.

Hiccough at the hour when the fever ought to come: [**Ars.**]

Nausea: Cough, d.: Ant-t, Ars, Bry, *Calc*, Hep, **Ipec,** *Merc*, **Puls,** *Sep*; **deathly:** *Ars*, **Ipec, Lob; fever,** a.: **Ars; drinking,** a.: Ant-t, *Ars*, Bry, Lyc, *Phos*, **Puls,** Rhus, Sil, >: **Bry,** *Lob*, *Phos*, **ice cream,** a.: *Ars*, *Ipec*, **Puls; odor** from his own body, at: [**Sulf**]; putting hands in hot **water,** on: [**Phos**]; **rising** up in bed, on: *Ars*, **Bry,** Phos, Sulf; **warm** drinks: **Phos, Puls;** warm room: Carb-v, **Lyc,** *Phos*, *Puls*, Sep.

Thirst: Noon: **Lyc,** Phos; 2 p. m.: [**Puls**]; **night: Sil; chill, b.: Ars,** *Hep,* **Puls,** Sep, Sulf, **d.:** *Acon,* Ars, *Bry, Calc, Carb-v,* Nat-s, *Rhus,* **Sep, Sil,** *Sulf,* **Tub, a.: Ars,** Hep, Nat-s, **Puls,** Sep, Sulf; **heat,** d.: **Acon, Ars, Bell, Bry,** *Calc, Hep, Ipec,* Lyc, *Phos, Puls, Rhus,* Sep, *Sil, Sulf,* **Tub;** for **large** quantities: *Acon,* **Ars, Bry,** *Ferr-p,* **Phos, Sulf,** often: **Bry,** at long intervals: [**Bry**]; **sweat,** d.: *Acon,* **Ars,** *Bry,* Calc, *Iod, Ipec,* Puls, *Rhus, Sep,* **a.:** *Ant-t,* Bell, **Lyc; small** quantities: Ant-t, **Ars,** Bell, **Lyc,** Phos, *Rhus, Sulf,* often: Acon, Ant-t, **Ars,** *Bell,* Lyc, Puls, Rhus, *Sulf.*

Thirstless: Heat, d.: *Ant-t, Calc, Carb-v, Ipec,* Lyc, *Puls,* Rhus, **Sep,** *Sulf.*

RESPIRATION

Abdominal: Ant-t, Bry, *Phos.*

Accelerated: Acon, Ant-t, Ars, Bell, Bry, Calc, **Carb-v, Chel,** *Hep, Iod,* **Ipec, Lyc,** *Merc,* **Phos,** *Puls, Rhus, Sang,* Seneg, **Sep,** *Sil,* **Sulf,** Tub, *Verat-v.*

Anxious: Acon, Ant-t, **Ars,** *Bell,* Bry, Calc, **Chel,** *Hep,* **Ipec,** Lob, **Phos, Puls,** *Rhus.*

Arrested: Ars, Bell, **Bry,** *Calc,* Carb-v, Iod, *Lyc,* Merc, Nat-s, *Phos, Puls,* Sep, *Sil, Sulf*; **night: Lyc; cough,** d.: *Acon,* **Ant-t, Ars,** Bell, Bry, Calc, Carb-v Hep, Iod, **Ipec,** Lob, *Lyc,* Merc, Nat-s, Phos, Puls, Rhus, Sang, *Sep, Sil,* Sulf.

Asphyxia: Ant-t, Carb-v, Rhus.

Catching: *Calc, Phos,* **Sil,** Sulf; night and d. fever: [**Sil**].

Deep: Desire to breathe: Acon, **Bry, Calc,** *Carb-v, Lyc, Merc,* **Nat-s,** *Phos, Sang, Seneg,* Sep, **Sulf; impossible: Ars,** Bry, *Lob,* Sulf.

Difficult: Evening: Acon, Ant-t, *Ars,* Bell, *Carb-v,* Ferr-p, Ipec, *Lob,* Merc, *Phos, Puls, Rhus,* Sep, **Sulf,** 6 p. m.: **Rhus; night:** Acon, *Ant-t,* **Ars,** Bell, Bry, *Calc, Carb-v,* Chel, *Ferr-p, Iod, Ipec, Lob, Lyc,* Merc,

Phos, *Puls*, *Rhus*, Seneg, *Sep*, **Sulf**, *Tub*, in bed: **Ars**, >: *Chel*; **midnight:** *Acon*, **Ars**, Calc, Puls, *Rhus*, **a.:** **Ars**, Lyc, 2 a. m.: **Ars**, 3 a. m.: **Ant-t**; **air**, cold: *Ars*, **Lob**, *Lyc*, *Merc*, Puls, Seneg, Sulf; **children:** Calc, Lyc, **Nat-s**, *Puls*; **cough**, d.: Acon, **Ant-t**, **Ars**, *Bell*, Bry, Calc, *Carb-v*, Ferr-p, *Hep*, **Ipec**, Lob, *Lyc*, Merc, *Nat-s*, **Phos**, Rhus, *Sep*, *Sil*, Sulf; **dust**, as from: **Ars**, Bell, *Calc*, *Hep*, Ipec, Phos, **Sil**, Sulf; **eating**, a.: Ars, Calc, *Carb-v*, Chel, Merc, **Phos**, **Puls**, Rhus, Sang, *Sulf*; > **eructations:** **Carb-v**; **exertion**, a.: **Ars**, **Calc**, *Carb-v*, *Iod*, **Ipec**, **Lob**, **Lyc**, *Merc*, *Nat-s*, *Phos*, *Puls*, Sep, *Sil*, *Sulf*; **expectoration** >: **Ant-t**, Ipec, *Sep*; **fanned**, desire to be: Ant-t, **Carb-v**, Sulf; **flatulence**, from: **Carb-v**, *Lyc*, *Nat-s*, Sang; **lying**, while: Acon, *Ant-t*, **Ars**, Calc, **Carb-v**, Ferr-p, *Hep*, **Lob**, *Lyc*, *Merc*, *Phos*, *Puls*, Sang, *Seneg*, *Sep*, *Sil*, *Sulf*, **Tub**, >: Bry, *Chel*, Nat-s, on back: *Ars*, *Iod*, **Lyc**, *Phos*, *Puls*, *Sil*, Sulf, impossible: *Ant-t*, **Ars**, *Hep*, *Lyc*, *Merc*, *Puls*, *Seneg*, *Sep*, *Sulf*, *Tub*; **menses** suppressed: **Puls**; **motion:** *Ars*, **Bry**, Calc, *Carb-v*, Iod, Ipec, *Lob*, *Lyc*, Merc, *Nat-s*, *Phos*, Puls, Rhus, *Sep*; **mucus** in trachea, from: **Ant-t**, **Ars**, *Ipec*; **open**, wants doors and windows: *Carb-v*, *Chel*, *Ipec*, *Nat-s*, **Puls**, **Sulf**; sulfur **fumes**, as if he had inhaled: **Lyc**, **Puls**, Sulf; **talking**, a.: *Ars*, Bry, *Sil*, **Sulf**; **turning** in bed, on: **Ars**, *Carb-v*, *Sulf*; **warm** room: Ant-t, Ars, *Carb-v*, *Iod*, Ipec, *Lyc*, **Puls**, **Sulf**, Tub; **wet** weather: **Nat-s**.

Gasping: *Acon*, *Ant-t*, *Ars*, *Ipec*, **Lyc**, Merc, *Phos*, Puls.

Hot breath: **Acon**, *Ars*, *Bell*, Calc, Chel, *Phos*, *Rhus*, *Sulf*.

Impeded: Flatulence, by: **Carb-v**; pain, by: **Bry**.

Intermittent, unequal: **Ant-t**, Bell.

Irregular: *Ant-t*, *Ars*, **Bell**, *Iod*, Merc, Phos, *Puls*, Sep, Verat-v.

Loud: Acon, Ant-t, Ars, **Calc**, *Carb-v*, *Hep*, Merc, *Nat-s*, **Phos**, *Puls*, *Rhus*, *Seneg*, **Sulf**; sleep, d.: Carb-v, **Puls**.

Panting: Acon, *Ant-t*, Ars, *Bry*, *Ipec*, *Lyc*, **Phos.** *Sil.* **Verat-v.**

Rattling: *Acon*, **Ant-t, Ars,** *Bell*, Bry, *Calc*, *Carb-v*, *Chel*, Ferr-p, **Hep,** *Iod*, **Ipec,** Lob, **Lyc,** Merc, *Nat-s*, **Phos, Puls,** *Sang*, **Seneg,** *Sep*, *Sil*, *Sulf*, *Tub*; **aged:** **Lyc,** *Seneg.*

Rough: *Ant-t*, **Bry,** *Hep*; crowing: **Bry;** sawing: *Ant-t*, **Iod,** *Sang.*

Sighing: *Acon*, *Ars*, Bell, **Bry,** *Calc*, **Carb-v, Ipec,** *Lyc*, *Phos*, *Puls*, Sang, Sil, Sulf, Verat-v.

Stertorous: Acon, *Ant-t*, *Ars*, Bell, *Lyc*, Phos, *Puls*, sleep, d.: **Puls.**

Stridulous: **Bell,** *Sang*; evening on falling asleep: [**Phos**].

Wheezing: **Ars,** Calc, **Carb-v,** Hep, *Iod*, **Ipec,** *Lyc*, Merc, *Nat-s*, Phos, Sang. Sep, Sulf.

COUGH

Daytime only: *Calc*, Hep, Lyc, Merc, *Phos*, Sep.

Morning: Acon, Ant-t, **Ars,** Bell, Bry, **Calc,** Carb-v, *Chel*, Ferr-p, Hep, *Iod*, Ipec, *Lyc*, Merc, Nat-s, **Phos, Puls,** Rhus, Sang, Seneg, *Sep*, *Sil*, **Sulf; rising,** a.: *Ars*, Bry, Calc, Carb-v, Ferr-p, Nat-s, **Phos,** Sep, *Sil*, Sulf; **waking:** Carb-v, *Chel*, Phos, Rhus, **Sil,** Sulf,

Evening: Acon, Ant-t, **Ars,** *Bell*, Bry, **Calc, Carb-v,** Chel, Ferr-p, **Hep,** Iod, Ipec, **Lyc, Merc,** *Phos*, Rhus, *Sang*, *Seneg*, *Sep*, Sil, Sulf, Verat-v; **bed,** in: Acon, Ant-t, **Ars,** Bell, *Calc*, *Carb-v*, **Hep,** Ipec, **Lyc, Merc,** *Phos*, *Puls*, Rhus, **Sep,** *Sil*, **Sulf; midnight,** until: Bell, Carb-v, **Hep,** Merc, **Phos,** *Puls*, *Rhus*, *Sep*, Sulf; **sleep,** going to: *Hep*, **Lyc.**

Night: **Acon,** Ant-t, **Ars, Bell,** Bry, **Calc,** Carb-v, *Chel*, *Ferr-p*, *Hep*, *Ipec*, **Lyc, Merc,** Nat-s, Phos, **Puls,** *Rhus*, *Sang*, Seneg, **Sep, Sil, Sulf; waking** from cough: *Bell*, *Calc*, Hep, Phos, *Puls*, Sang, **Sep,** Sil, **Sulf; midnight,** b.: Ant-t, Ars, Bell, Calc, **Carb-v,** Hep, *Lyc*, *Phos*, Puls, Rhus, Sep, Sulf.

Air: Cold: Acon, **Ars,** Bry, *Calc*, *Carb-v*, Ferr-p, **Hep,** Ipec, Lyc, Nat-s, **Phos,** *Rhus*, Sang, *Seneg*, *Sep*. Sil, Sulf, Verat-v, dry: **Acon, Hep,** *Phos*; **open:** *Acon*, **Ars,** Bry, Calc, Carb-v, Ferr-p, *Hep*, Ipec, Lyc, **Phos,** *Rhus*, Sang, Seneg, Sil, *Sulf*, >: **Bry,** Chel, **Iod,** *Nat-s*, **Puls,** Sulf.

Barking: **Acon,** Ant-t, **Bell, Hep,** Lyc, Merc, Phos, Sulf; **loud:** **Acon,** Lyc.

Bathing <: Ars, *Calc*, **Rhus,** Sep, Sulf.

Bed, on becoming warm in < or excites: Ant-t, Merc, **Puls.**

Breathing deeply: *Acon*, Ars, **Bell, Bry,** Ferr-p, *Hep*, *Iod*, Ipec, *Lyc*, *Merc*, Phos, *Puls*, *Rhus*, Seneg, Sep, Sil, *Sulf*.

Chill: B.: **Rhus,** *Tub*; **d.:** Acon, *Ars*, Bell, *Bry*, Calc, Carb-v, Hep, Ipec. Lyc, **Phos,** *Puls*, **Rhus,** *Sep*, Sil, Sulf, *Tub*.

Choking: Ars, Carb-v, *Hep*, Iod, **Ipec,** Lyc, Merc, *Sep*, *Sulf*.

Closing eyes at night excites cough: [**Hep**].

Cold: Becoming: **Ars,** *Bry*, *Calc*, *Carb-v*, **Hep, Phos, Rhus,** *Sang*, **Sil,** *Sulf*, **Tub,** arm or hand: Ars, Calc, **Hep, Rhus,** *Sil*, Sulf, feet: *Sil*, Sulf, single part: **Hep, Rhus,** Sil; **drinks:** **Ars,** Calc, *Carb-v*, *Hep*, Lyc, *Merc*, *Phos*, Rhus, *Sil*, *Tub*.

Constant: Acon, Ant-t, *Ars*, Bell, Bry, Calc, *Carb-v*, Ferr-p, *Hep*, *Ipec*, **Lyc,** Merc, Phos, *Puls*, *Rhus*, Sang, *Seneg*, Sep; **evening:** Acon, **Puls; night:** Lyc **Sep,** lying down: **Sep,** waking: [**Sep**]; **lying** <, **sitting** up >: **Puls,** Rhus, Sang, **Sep.**

Constriction of larynx: *Ant-t*, *Ars*, *Bell*. *Calc*, *Hep*, *Iod*, *Ipec*, *Lob*, **Phos,** *Puls*, *Sil*, *Sulf*.

Crawling sense in throat-pit causes: **Sang.**

Croupy: **Acon,** Ant-t, *Ars*, *Bell*, **Hep, Iod,** *Ipec*, **Phos,** *Sang*.

Drinking: A.: Acon, Ant-t, **Ars,** *Bry*, Calc, Carb-v, *Hep*, Lyc, *Phos*, Rhus, Sil.

Dry: Acon, Ant-t, **Ars, Bell, Bry, Calc,** *Carb-v, Chel, Ferr-p, Hep,* **Iod,** *Ipec,* Lob, *Lyc, Merc,* Nat-s, **Phos, Puls,** *Rhus, Sang, Seneg, Sep, Sil,* **Sulf, Tub,** Verat-v; **morning:** Ant-t, Bry, *Carb-v,* Hep, **Iod,** Lyc, Nat-s, *Rhus,* Sang, Sep, Sil, Sulf; **evening:** *Ars, Bell,* Bry, *Calc,* Carb-v, **Hep, Lyc,** Merc, *Phos,* **Puls,** *Rhus, Sang, Seneg, Sep,* **Sulf,** loose mornings: Acon, Ant-t, *Bry,* **Calc,** *Carb-v,* **Hep,** Ipec, Lyc, *Phos, Puls,* Rhus, Seneg, *Sep, Sil,* Sulf, lying down: *Bell,* Carb-v, **Puls, Sang, Sep, Sulf; night:** Acon, **Ars, Bell,** Bry, **Calc,** *Carb-v, Chel,* **Hep,** *Ipec, Lyc, Merc,* Nat-s, **Phos, Puls,** *Rhus, Sang, Sil,* **Sulf,** loose by day: Acon, Ars, Bry, *Calc, Hep, Lyc,* Merc, Phos, *Puls,* Sil, **Sulf,** lying<: *Puls,* **Sulf,**> sitting up: **Puls,** Sang, waking from sleep: *Puls, Sil,* **Sulf,** b. **midnight: Calc,** *Lyc,* Phos, Rhus; **chill,** b.: **Rhus,** *Tub;* expectoration morning only: Bell, *Bry, Calc, Carb-v, Hep,* Lyc, *Phos,* **Puls,** *Sep, Sil;* **fever,** d.: **Acon,** *Ars,* Bell, **Bry,** Calc, Carb-v, Hep, **Ipec,** Lyc, **Phos,** Puls, Rhus, Sep, Sulf;> sitting up and passing **flatus** up and down: [**Sang**]; **lying:** Ipec, Lyc, Phos, **Puls,** Rhus, *Sang,* Sep, Sil, Sulf, on l. side<: Acon, Bry, **Phos,** Puls; **reading** aloud: **Phos; scraping** in larynx, from: *Bell,* Bry, Chel, **Puls,** Seneg; **stomach,** as if from: **Bry, Sep; tickling** in larynx, from: *Bell,* Iod, **Ipec, Lyc,** Nat-s, **Puls,** *Sang, Seneg, Sep;* **waking,** on: Bry, Calc, *Puls, Sang,* Sil, **Sulf.**

Dryness in larynx, from: Ant-t, Bell, Bry, *Calc,* Ipec, *Puls,* Rhus, **Sang,** Seneg, *Sulf,* Verat-v.

Dust, as from: **Ars,** *Bell, Calc,* Chel, *Hep,* Iod, *Ipec,* **Lyc, Puls, Sulf.**

Eructations>: [Sang].

Exertion, from: Bry, Iod, Ipec, *Lyc,* Merc, Phos, **Puls,** Sil, Sulf.

Exhausting: Ant-t, **Ars, Bell,** *Carb-v,* Chel, Ferr-p, Iod, *Ipec,* Lyc, *Merc, Phos, Puls, Rhus,* Sang, Seneg, **Sep,** *Sil,* Sulf; **night: Puls,** disturbing sleep: [**Puls**].

Fever, d.: **Acon,** Ant-t, **Ars,** *Bell, Bry,* **Calc,** Carb-v, Ferr-p, Hep, Iod, **Ipec,** Lyc, **Phos,** Puls, Rhus, Sang, Seneg, Sep, Sil, Sulf, *Tub.*

Flatus, passing>: [**Sang**].

Foreign body, as of a, larynx: **Bell,** *Hep,* Lob, *Phos, Sil;* trachea: **Sang.**

Hacking: Acon, Ant-t, **Ars,** *Bry, Calc,* Carb-v, Ferr-p, Hep, Ipec, Lyc, Merc, **Phos,** *Rhus,* **Sang,** *Seneg,* **Sep,** *Sil, Sulf,* **Tub,** Verat-v; **afternoon: Sang; evening:** Bry, Phos, *Rhus,* **Sang, Sep,** Sil, *Sulf,* in bed: Bry, *Rhus,* **Sep,** *Sulf,* a. lying down: *Rhus,* **Sang, Sep,** Sil; **dinner,** a.: **Hep; dryness** in larynx, from: *Puls,* **Sang,** *Seneg;* **lying** down, while: *Ars, Bry,* Phos, Rhus, **Sang,** Sep, Sil, Sulf; **tickling** in larynx, from: Acon, **Ars,** *Bry, Calc,* Carb-v, Ipec, Lyc, **Phos,** Rhus, *Sang, Seneg,* Sep, Sil.

Hoarse: Acon, Ant-t, **Bell,** *Calc,* **Carb-v, Hep,** *Lyc,* Merc, *Rhus, Sil;* evening until midnight: [**Hep**].

Hold chest with hands, must: **Bry,** Merc, *Nat-s, Phos, Sep.*

Hollow: *Acon,* Ant-t, **Bell,** Bry, Carb-v, Chel, Hep, *Ipec,* Merc, *Phos,* Sil.

Irritation: Air passages: **Acon,** Ant-t, *Calc, Carb-v,* Ferr-p, **Iod,** Lob, Lyc, Nat-s, Phos, **Sep,** *Sulf;* **chest:** Ars, *Bell, Calc, Carb-v, Ferr-p,* Merc, **Phos,** Puls, Rhus, *Sang,* **Sep; epigastrium:** Bell, **Bry,** *Hep,* Merc, **Puls, Sep; larynx:** *Acon,* Ant-t, Ars, **Bell,** *Bry, Calc, Carb-v,* Chel, **Hep,** *Iod,* **Ipec,** *Lyc, Merc,* **Phos, Puls,** *Rhus,* Sang, *Seneg, Sep, Sil,* **Sulf; throat-pit:** Bell, Iod, **Sang,** *Sil;* **trachea:** Acon, Ant-t, Ars, *Bell, Bry, Calc, Carb-v, Ferr-p,* Hep, *Iod,* Ipec, **Lyc,** *Merc,* **Phos,** *Puls,* **Rhus,** Seneg, **Sep, Sil, Sulf.**

Loose: Ant-t, **Ars,** Bell, Bry, *Calc, Carb-v, Chel,* Ferr-p, Hep, Iod, Lyc, Merc, Nat-s, *Phos,* **Puls,** Seneg, *Sep, Sil,* Sulf, Verat-v; **morning:** Ars, **Bry,** *Calc,* **Carb-v,** *Chel,* **Hep,** Nat-s, *Phos,* **Puls, Sep,** *Sil,* **Sulf; fever,** d.: **Ars,** Bell, Bry, **Calc,** Carb-v, Iod, Lyc, Phos, Puls, Seneg, Sep, *Sil, Sulf.*

Lying: <: Acon, Ant-t, *Ars*, Bell, *Bry*, Calc, *Carb-v*, Ferr-p, Hep, *Iod*, Ipec, *Lyc*, Merc, Nat-s, *Phos*, **Puls**, *Rhus*, **Sang**, *Seneg*, *Sep*, *Sil*, *Sulf*; **evening:** *Bell*, Bry, **Puls**, **Sang**, *Seneg*, **Sep**, *Sil*, *Sulf*, must sit up: **Ars**, **Puls**, **Sang**, **Sep**; **night:** *Ars*, *Bell*, Lyc, Nat-s, **Puls**, Rhus, **Sang**, **Sep**, Sil, Sulf; **bed** <**:** Ant-t, *Ars*, Bry, Calc, Ferr-p, Hep, Iod, Ipec, Lyc, **Phos**, *Puls*, *Rhus*, Sang, *Sep*, *Sil*, **Sulf**; r. **side:** Ipec, Lyc, **Merc**, Phos, Sil, Tub.

Mucus in chest, from: Ant-t, Ars, *Calc*, Iod, Ipec, **Puls**, Sep, Sulf.

Overpowering, as if larynx were tickled by a feather, evening b. sleep: [**Lyc**].

Painful: Ant-t, **Bry**, Ferr-p, *Merc*, Nat-s, Rhus.

Paroxysmal: Acon, *Ars*, **Bell**, Bry, *Calc*, **Carb-v**, *Chel*, Ferr-p, **Hep**, Iod, **Ipec**, Lob, Lyc, Merc, Phos, **Puls**, Sang, *Seneg*, **Sep**, Sil, *Sulf*; **night:** Ant-t, **Bell**, Bry, Calc, **Carb-v**, *Chel*, *Hep*, *Ipec*, Lyc, *Merc*, *Phos*, *Puls*, Sang, Sil, Sulf.

Persistent: Acon, **Bell**, Ipec, Lyc, Merc, Sang.

Racking: Ars, **Bell**, **Bry**, Calc, **Carb-v**, *Chel*, *Ipec*, *Lyc*, **Merc**, **Phos**, **Puls**, *Rhus*, *Seneg*, *Sep*, *Sil*, **Sulf**; **night:** **Bell**, Merc; > **sitting** up: **Puls**.

Rattling: **Ant-t**, *Bell*, *Bry*, *Calc*, *Carb-v*, *Chel*, Ferr-p, *Hep*, *Iod*, **Ipec**, *Lyc*, Merc, *Nat-s*, Phos, *Puls*, *Sang*, **Sep**, *Sil*, *Sulf*, Verat-v.

Rawness in larynx excites: Acon, *Bry*, *Hep*, **Phos**, Sang, *Sil*, **Sulf**.

Reading aloud: <: **Phos**, *Tub*; evening: *Phos*.

Scraping in larynx, from: *Bell*, *Bry*, **Carb-v**, Chel, **Hep**, **Puls**, *Seneg*, Sil.

Short: **Acon**, Ant-t, *Ars*, *Bell*, *Bry*, *Calc*, Carb-v, *Chel*, Ferr-p, Hep, Iod, Ipec, Lob, *Lyc*, *Merc*, *Phos*, Puls, **Rhus**, Seneg, **Sep**, Sulf, Verat-v.

Sit up, must: *Ant-t*, *Ars*, *Bry*, Hep, *Iod*, Nat-s, **Phos**, **Puls**, *Sang*, *Seneg*, *Sep*.

Sleep: B.: Lyc, Merc, **Sulf; disturbing:** Phos, Rhus, Sang, **Sulf;** going to, on: *Carb-v*, *Hep*, **Lyc,** Merc, *Phos*, Sep, **Sulf; preventing:** Carb-v, **Lyc,** Phos, **Puls,** *Rhus*, Sang, **Sep; wakens** from: Acon, *Ars*, Bell, Calc, Hep, Merc, **Phos,** *Rhus*, *Sang*, *Sep*, *Sil*, **Sulf.**

Spasmodic: Acon, *Ars*, **Bell, Bry,** *Calc*, **Carb-v,** *Chel*, Ferr-p, *Hep*, *Iod*, **Ipec,** *Lob*, Lyc, *Merc*, *Phos*, **Puls,** *Rhus*, *Sang*, **Sep,** Sil, *Sulf*, Verat-v; **afternoon: Bell,** Bry; **evening:** Bell Bry, Calc, *Carb-v*, *Ipec*, Merc, *Phos*, *Puls*, Rhus, **Sep,** Sil, Verat-v; **night: Bell,** *Bry*, Calc, *Hep*, *Ipec*, Lyc, Merc, *Phos*, *Puls*, *Sang*, Sil, Sulf.

Stomach, seems to come from: Ant-t, Bell, **Bry,** Merc, Puls, **Sep.**

Suffocative: Acon, *Ant-t*, *Ars*, Bell, *Bry*, **Carb-v,** Chel, **Hep,** *Iod*, **Ipec,** Lyc, *Merc*, *Puls*, *Sep*, Sil, **Sulf,** *Tub*; **7 p. m.:** [**Ipec**]; **night:** Ars, Bell, Bry, *Carb-v*, **Hep,** Ipec, Lyc, Sil; **child** becomes stiff and blue in face: **Ipec.**

Sulfur fumes, as from: <: **Ars,** Bry, Calc, *Carb-v*, Ipec, **Lyc, Puls.**

Tickling: Acon, Ant-t, Ars, *Bell*, *Bry*, *Calc*, *Carb-v*, *Ferr-p*, Hep, *Iod*, **Ipec, Lyc,** Merc, *Phos*, *Puls*, *Rhus*, **Sang,** *Seneg*, **Sep,** Sil, Sulf; **air,** open: **Phos**; in **chest:** Bry, Iod, *Merc*, **Phos,** Rhus, Sep, Sulf, Verat-v; in **larynx:** *Acon*, Ant-t, **Ars, Bell,** *Bry*, *Calc*, *Carb-v*, *Chel*, *Hep*, **Iod, Ipec,** Lob, **Lyc,** Merc, Nat-s, **Phos, Puls,** Rhus, *Sang*, *Seneg*, *Sep*, *Sil*, Sulf; **throat-pit;** Bell, Iod, Puls, **Sang,** *Sil*; **trachea:** *Acon*, *Ant-t*, Ars, Bell, Bry, *Calc*, **Iod,** *Merc*, *Phos*, *Puls*, **Rhus, Sang,** *Seneg*, *Sep*, **Sil,** Sulf.

Tight: Merc, **Phos,** *Puls*, *Sulf*.

Tormenting: Ars, Bell, *Calc*, Carb-v, Chel, Ferr-p, Hep, **Ipec,** Lob, Merc, *Phos*, Rhus, *Sang*, Sep, *Sulf*.

Uncovering: <: Ars, Chel, **Hep, Rhus,** Sil, feet or head: [**Sil**], hands: **Hep, Rhus,** Sil.

Violent: Ant-t, Ars, **Bell,** Bry, *Calc*, **Carb-v,** *Chel*, **Hep, Ipec,** *Lob*, *Merc*, **Phos, Puls,** *Rhus*, Sang, Seneg, **Sep,** *Sil*, Sulf; **evening** a. lying: **Sep.**

Warm fluids>: **Ars,** *Bry,* **Lyc, Rhus, Sil; room** causes: Acon, Ars, *Bry, Iod, Ipec, Lyc,* Phos, **Puls,** *Seneg,* Sulf, *Tub.*

Wind<: *Acon,* **Hep,** Lyc, Sep; **cold: Hep,** Lyc, dry; **Acon, Hep; east: Acon, Hep,** Sep; **north: Acon, Hep,** Sep, **west:** [**Hep**].

EXPECTORATION

Daytime: Acon, Ant-t, **Ars,** *Bell,* Bry, *Calc,* Ferr-p, **Hep,** *Lyc,* **Merc,** Phos, **Puls,** Rhus, **Sil, Sulf.**

Morning: Acon, *Ant-t,* Ars, Bell, **Bry,** *Calc,* **Carb-v,** *Ferr-p,* **Hep,** Iod, Ipec, Lyc, Nat-s, **Phos, Puls,** *Rhus,* Seneg, **Sep, Sil, Sulf; rising:** *Phos,* **Puls.**

Night: Ars, Calc, Carb-v, Hep, Lyc, Phos, Puls, Rhus, **Sep,** Sil, Sulf.

Bloody: Acon, Ars, *Bell, Bry, Calc, Carb-v,* **Ferr-p,** Hep, Iod, **Ipec,** *Lyc, Merc,* **Phos, Puls,** *Rhus,* Sang, *Sep, Sil,* **Sulf; acrid:** *Ars,* Carb-v, Hep, Rhus, **Sil,** Sulf; **bright** red: **Acon,** Ars, **Bell,** Bry, *Calc, Carb-v,* Ferr-p, *Ipec, Merc, Phos,* Puls, *Rhus,* Sep, Sil; **brown: Bry,** *Calc,* **Carb-v,** Puls, *Rhus,* Sil; **streaked:** *Acon,* **Ars, Bry,** Calc, *Chel,* Hep, Iod, *Ipec, Lyc,* Merc, *Phos,* Puls, Sang, Seneg, Sep, Sil.

Copious: Ant-t, **Ars,** Bry, **Calc,** *Carb-v, Chel,* Ferr-p, **Hep,** *Iod,* Lob, **Lyc, Phos, Puls,** *Seneg,* **Sep,** *Sil, Sulf.*

Difficult: *Ars,* Bry, *Calc, Chel,* Ferr-p, *Hep,* **Ipec,** *Iod,* Lob, Lyc, *Phos,* **Puls, Seneg,** Sep, Sulf.

Frothy: *Acon,* Ant-t, **Ars,** Calc, Ferr-p, Hep, *Phos, Puls,* Sil, Sulf.

Grayish: *Ars, Calc,* Chel, Iod, **Lyc,** *Phos,* Rhus, *Seneg, Sep.*

Greenish: *Ars,* Bry, *Calc,* **Carb-v,** *Ferr-p,* Iod, **Lyc, Merc, Nat-s, Phos, Puls,** Rhus, *Sep, Sil,* **Sulf,** *Tub.*

Lumpy: Acon, Ars, Bry, Carb-v, Chel, *Hep,* Lyc, Phos, Puls, **Sil,** Sulf.

Mucus: Acon, *Ant-t*, **Ars**, Bell, **Bry**, **Calc**, *Carb-v*, Chel, Ferr-p, **Hep**, *Iod*, Ipec, **Lob**, **Lyc**, Merc, *Nat-s*, **Phos**, **Puls**, *Rhus*, **Sang**, *Seneg*, *Sep*, **Sil**, Sulf; **morning:** *Ant-t*, Bell, *Calc*, Chel, Ipec, Lyc, *Phos*, Puls, Sil, **Sulf**; **bloody:** *Acon*, Ant-t, **Ars**, Bell, *Bry*, *Calc*, Hep, Iod, **Ipec**, Lyc, *Merc*, **Phos**, Sil.

Odor offensive: **Ars**, Bell, Bry, **Calc**, Carb-v, Ferr-p, Hep, Iod, **Lyc**, Merc, Puls, *Rhus*, **Sang**, Seneg, *Sep*, *Sil*, Sulf.

Purulent: Acon, *Ant-t*, *Ars*, Bell, Bry, **Calc**, Carb-v, Ferr-p, Hep, Iod, Ipec, **Lyc**, *Merc*, Nat-s, **Phos**, *Puls*, *Rhus*, Sang, **Sep**, **Sil**, *Sulf*.

Rusty: *Acon*, *Ars*, **Bry**, **Lyc**, *Phos*, *Rhus*, *Sang*.

Scanty: Acon, Ars, Ferr-p, Lyc, **Phos**, *Puls*, Sang, Sep, Sil.

Taste: Bitter: Acon, *Ars*, Bry, Calc, Lyc, *Merc*, **Puls**, *Sep*, Sulf; **catarrh**, as of an old: *Bell*, Phos, **Puls**, *Sulf*; **greasy:** Lyc, Phos, **Puls**, Rhus, *Sil*; **nauseous:** *Ars*, Bry, Calc, Iod, *Ipec*, *Merc*, Phos, **Puls**, Sep, Sil, Sulf; **salty:** Acon, Ant-t, **Ars**, Bell, *Calc*, *Carb-v*, Iod, **Lyc**, *Merc*, **Phos**, **Puls**, Rhus, **Sep**, Sil, Sulf; **sour:** Ant-t, Ars, *Bell*, Bry, **Calc**, Carb-v, Hep, Iod, Ipec, Lyc, *Merc*, **Phos**, *Puls*, Rhus, Sep, *Sulf*; **sweetish:** Acon, Ant-t, Ars, **Calc**, Hep, Iod, Ipec, Lyc, Merc, **Phos**, *Puls*, Rhus, Sep, Sulf.

Thick: Acon, Ant-t, *Ars*, Bry, *Calc*, Ferr-p, **Hep**, Ipec, *Lyc*, Phos, *Puls*, Sang, Seneg, *Sep*, **Sil**, Sulf, **Tub.**

Tough: Acon, *Ant-t*, *Ars*, Bell, *Bry*, **Calc**, Carb-v, **Hep**, *Iod*, Phos, Puls, Sang, Seneg, *Sep*, Sil.

Transparent: Ant-t, *Ars*, Bry, **Phos**, Puls, **Seneg**, *Sil*, Sulf.

Viscid: Acon, Ant-t, *Ars*, Bell, *Bry*, *Calc*, *Carb-v*, Ferr-p, **Hep**, *Iod*, Lyc, Merc, **Phos**, **Puls**, Rhus, Sang, **Seneg**, *Sep*, *Sil*, Sulf.

White: *Acon*, Ant-t, *Ars*, *Calc*, *Carb-v*, Ferr-p, *Iod*, Ipec, **Lyc**, **Phos**, *Puls*, Rhus, Sang, **Seneg**, **Sep**, Sil, *Sulf*; **albuminous:** Ant-t, *Ars*, Bry, Ipec, *Nat-s*, **Phos**, **Seneg**, *Sil*, Sulf.

Yellow: *Acon*, *Ars*, Bell, *Bry*, **Calc**, *Carb-v*, *Ferr-p*, **Hep**, Iod, Ipec, **Lyc**, *Merc*, **Phos**, **Puls**, Sang, Seneg, **Sep**, **Sil**, *Sulf*, **Tub**; **morning:** *Calc*, Lyc, *Phos*, **Puls**, *Sil*.

CHEST

Abscess: Lungs: **Calc**, **Hep**, *Lyc*, *Merc*, **Phos**, *Puls*, Sep, **Sil**, *Sulf*, *Tub*.

Anxiety in: **Acon**, **Ars**, Bell, *Bry*, **Calc**, *Carb-v*, *Chel*, Ferr-p, Iod, *Ipec*, *Lob*, *Lyc*, **Merc**, **Phos**, *Puls*, Rhus, Seneg, Sep, *Sulf*; **evening:** Chel, *Phos*, **Puls**, Seneg; **night:** *Ars*, Lyc, **Puls**, Sulf; **excitement** <: [**Phos**]; **lying** on l. side, while: [**Puls**]; region of **heart:** **Acon**, **Ant-t**, **Ars**, **Bell**, *Calc*, **Carb-v**, Chel, Ferr-p, *Iod*, **Ipec**, Lob, *Lyc*, *Merc*, **Phos**, *Puls*, *Rhus*, Sep, Sil, Sulf, **night:** **Ars**, Calc, Lyc, Rhus.

Atelectasis: **Ant-t**.

Coldness: **Ars**, Bry, Lyc, Rhus, Sep, **Sulf**; int.: **Ars**, *Sulf*.

Congestion: **Acon**, **Bell**, **Bry**, *Calc*, *Carb-v*, Ferr-p, *Iod*, **Ipec**, *Lyc*, *Merc*, **Phos**, *Puls*, **Rhus**, *Seneg*, **Sep**, *Sil*, **Sulf**, *Verat-v*; **heart:** **Acon**, *Puls*, Sulf.

Constriction, tension, tightness: **Acon**, *Ant-t*, **Ars**, **Bell**, **Bry**, **Calc**, **Carb-v**, **Chel**, Ferr-p, *Hep*, *Iod*, *Ipec*, **Lob**, **Lyc**, *Merc*, **Phos**, *Puls*, *Rhus*, **Seneg**, *Sep*, **Sil**, **Sulf**; **band**, as from a: **Acon**, *Ars*, Bry, *Lob*, *Lyc*, **Phos**, Sil; **convulsive:** **Bell**; **cough**, d.: Calc, Lyc, Merc, **Phos**, *Puls*, *Sulf*; **sternum** on coughing: [**Phos**]; **heart:** **Ars**, Calc, Ferr-p, **Iod**, Lyc, Phos, Rhus, grasped, as if: **Iod**, Rhus.

Emphysema: **Ant-t**, *Ars*, *Bell*, *Carb-v*, **Hep**, *Ipec*, **Lob**, *Merc*, *Phos*, Seneg, Sep, Sulf.

Empyema: **Ars**, *Calc*, *Carb-v*, *Hep*, Iod, Lyc, **Merc**, *Phos*, *Sep*, **Sil**, **Sulf**.

Fullness: **Acon**, *Ars*, Bry, Calc, *Ferr-p*, *Lob*, Lyc, Merc, *Phos*, *Puls*, *Rhus*, Sang, Sep, *Sulf*; **evening:** *Carb-v*, **Puls**, *Sulf*; **menses**, b.: **Sulf**; **heart:** *Acon*, *Puls*, Sep, **Sulf**, evening: [**Puls**].

Gangrene, lungs: **Ars,** *Carb-v, Phos.*

Hemorrhage: **Acon,** *Ant-t,* **Ars,** *Bell, Bry, Calc,* Carb-v, **Chel,** Ferr-p, **Ipec,** Lyc, Merc, *Phos, Puls, Rhus, Sang,* Sep, Sil, Sulf; **coagulated:** Acon, *Bell,* Bry, *Ipec, Merc, Puls,* **Rhus,** Sep.

Heat: **Acon,** *Ant-t, Ars,* **Bell,** *Bry, Calc,* Ferr-p, *Hep,* Iod, *Lyc,* Merc, **Phos,** Puls, Rhus, *Seneg, Sep,* Sil, **Sulf;** **flushes:** *Phos,* **Seneg,** *Sep,* **Sulf,** rising to face: [**Sulf**], in region of **heart:** Ars, Carb-v, Lyc, **Phos,** Sep, Sil, *Sulf.*

Hepatization, lungs: Ant-t, *Chel, Iod, Lob, Lyc,* Merc, **Phos,** *Sang,* **Sulf,** *Tub;* **r.:** *Phos,* upper half. *Chel;* **l.:** *Lyc,* Phos, *Sulf;* lying on r. side>, on left<: [**Phos**].

Oppression: **Acon,** *Ant-t,* **Ars,** **Bell,** **Bry,** **Calc,** **Carb-v,** Chel, Ferr-p, *Hep, Iod,* **Ipec,** *Lob, Lyc, Merc,* **Nat-s,** **Phos,** **Puls,** *Rhus, Sang,* **Seneg,** **Sep,** *Sil,* **Sulf,** **Tub,** Verat-v; **morning:** *Ars,* Bry, Carb-v, Chel, *Ipec,* Lyc, *Nat-s, Phos, Puls,* **Sep,** *Sulf;* **evening:** Ars, *Bry, Phos,* **Puls,** Seneg, **Sep,** Sulf;> open **air:** Chel, **Puls,** Sep; when weather changes to **cold:** [**Ars**]; **clothing<:** **Ars,** **Chel,** Phos, *Sep;* **cough,** d.: *Ars,* **Phos,** *Seneg, Sil,* **Sulf;>** drawing shoulders back: [**Calc**];> **eructations:** **Carb-v,** **Lyc,** *Phos;* in **stormy** weather: [**Ars**]; **heart:** *Acon,* Ant-t, **Ars,** Bell, Bry, *Carb-v, Iod,* **Ipec,** *Merc, Nat-s, Phos,* **Puls,** evening: **Puls,** sitting: **Nat-s.**

PAIN: Ars, Bell, Bry, Phos, Seneg; **night:** Ars; **cough,** d.: Bell, Bry, Carb-v, Lyc, Phos, Puls, Seneg, Sulf; a. pneumonia: Lyc, Phos, Sulf; **inspirtion,** d.: Acon, Bry, Calc; **lying** on painful side, while: Bell,>: Bry, on sound side: Puls, on l. side: Phos, on r. side: Merc; < **motion:** Bell, Bry, Calc; >**pressure:** Bry; **respiration,** d., and if deep: Bry; **rising** up in bed, on: Phos; **sneezing,** on: Bry;> **warmth:** Phos; in middle of chest > pressure of hand: Bry; in **Sides:** Lyc, Sulf, r.: Bell, Chel, apex of r. lung: Ars, l.: Phos, in s. at 4 p. m.: Lyc, d. cough: Bry, Merc, Sulf, d. inspiration: Bry, Chel, laughing: Bry, lying on l. side: Phos, on motion: Bry: Chel, d. respiration and deep: Bry; in **Lower:** Puls, l.: Phos, while lying on l. side: Phos; in **Lungs:** Phos, l. and lower l.: Phos, above l. nipple: Sulf, apex, of r.: Ars; **Sternum** and behind on coughing: Bry, behind: Sang; in **Heart:** Acon, Ars, Puls, Rhus, evening: Puls, ext. to back: Sulf.

Aching: Sternum: Bry.

Burning: Ars, Carb-v; cough, d., and if dry: Iod, ext. to face: Sulf; **Sides:** R.: Bry, L: Phos.

Clawing: Seneg.

Cutting: Chill, a.: Acon; inspiration and motion, d.: Bry; **Heart:** Ars, Sulf.

Pressing: Seneg, Sulf; cough, d.: Bry; **Diaphragm:** Ipec; **Sternum:** Ars, Phos; **Heart:** Ars, evening: Puls.

Rawness: Lyc, Phos; cold air: Phos.

Sore, bruised: Bry, Calc, Chel, Hep, Phos, Puls, Seneg; coughing, from: Bry, Carb-v, Phos, Seneg, hold chest with hands: Bry; inspiring, on: Bry; > sitting upright: Bry; below Clavicle: Puls; **Sides:** R.: Chel; under **Sternum** on coughing: Bry.

Sticking in short ribs: Sep.

Stitching: Acon, Bry, Calc, Phos, Seneg, Sulf; chill, d.: Bry; coughing: Bell, Bry, Iod, Merc; fever, d.: Bry, inspiring: Acon, Bry; lying on l. side: Phos, > lying on painful side: Bry; < motion: Bry, >: Rhus; > pressure: Bry; respiration, d., and if deep: Bry; < sneezing: Merc; wandering: Puls; ext. to back: Sulf; **Anterior** part and on coughing: Merc; under r. **Clavicle:** Ars, Clavicle to scapula: Sulf; **Sides:** Bry, R.: Ars, Bry, Chel, apex: Ars, respiration, d.: Bry, to scapula: Sulf; L.: Phos, Seneg, Sulf, on inspiration: Sulf, > lying on r. side: Phos, ext. to back and scapula: Sulf, in Sides: nights: Lyc, on coughing: Bry, Merc, d. inspiration: Bry, Sulf, > lying on painful side: Bry, d. motion: Bry, lower r.: Chel, < motion: Bry; **Sternum:** Ars, d. cough: Bry; Heart: Bry, Sulf, to l. scapula: Sulf.

Palpitation: **Acon,** *Ant-t,* **Ars,** *Bell, Bry,* **Calc,** *Carb-v, Chel, Ferr-p, Hep,* **Iod,** Ipec, *Lob,* **Lyc, Merc. Phos, Puls,** *Rhus,* Sang, Seneg, **Sep,** *Sil,* **Sulf,** *Verat-v*; **daytime: Acon,** *Iod,* Rhus; **morning:** Chel, Lyc, **Phos,** *Rhus,* Sulf; **evening:** Carb-v, Chel, *Hep, Lyc,* **Phos,** Sep, Sil, *Sulf,* in bed: Calc, **Lyc,** *Phos, Sep, Sulf;* **night:** *Ars,* **Calc,** Ferr-p, *Iod, Lyc, Merc, Phos,* **Puls,** Sep, Sil, *Sulf,* in bed: *Iod,* **Puls,** *Rhus,* **Sulf; 3 a. m.: Ars; anxiety: Acon,** Ant-t, **Ars,** *Bry,* **Calc,** Carb-v, *Chel,* Ferr-p, *Hep, Iod,* Ipec, *Lyc, Merc,* **Phos, Puls,** *Rhus, Sep,* **Sulf; digestion,** d.: **Lyc,** *Sep;* **eating,** a.: *Acon,* **Calc,** *Carb-v,* Hep, **Lyc,** Merc, Phos, **Puls,** *Sep,* Sil, Sulf; **excitement,** a.: *Ars, Bell,* Calc, **Phos,** *Puls,* Seneg, *Sep;* **exertion: Ars, Calc,** Carb-v, Ferr-p, **Iod,** *Merc,* **Phos,** *Puls, Rhus,* Sil, *Sulf;* **fever,** d.: *Acon,* **Ars, Calc,** Merc, Phos, **Puls,** *Sep,* Sulf; **fright,** a.: **Acon,** *Puls;* **irregular: Ars,** *Chel,* Merc; **lying:** Chel, Lyc, **Puls,** *Rhus,* **Sulf,** on r. side:> **Phos,** on l. side, from: Bry, *Lyc,* **Phos, Puls,** Sep; **motion:** Acon, Bell, *Calc, Carb-v,* Ferr-p, Iod, Merc, **Phos,** *Sil,* Sulf, of arms: *Acon,* Bry, Chel, *Puls, Rhus,* Seneg, **Sulf,** least: *Carb-v, Merc,* **Phos; rising** from bed: Ars, **Phos,** or seat: **Phos; falling asleep:** *Calc, Carb-v,* Phos, Sil, **Sulf; stool,** a.: **Ars; supper,** a.: *Lyc,* **Puls; turning** in bed: *Lyc, Phos,* **Sulf; waking:** Acon, *Ars, Calc,* Hep, **Phos,** Rhus, *Sep, Sil.*

Paralysis, lungs: **Ant-t,** *Ars, Calc,* **Carb-v,** *Iod,* **Lyc,** *Phos*; old people: *Ant-t, Ars, Carb-v,* Lyc, Phos.

Pulsation: Bell, Calc, Chel, Lyc, Merc, *Phos, Puls,* **Seneg,** *Sep, Sil,* Sulf; **night: Puls,** interrupting sleep; [**Puls**], on **waking:** [**Sulf**].

Shocks: Ant-t, Calc, Hep, **Lyc,** Rhus, Sep, *Sulf;* cough, d.: **Lyc,** *Seneg.*

Ulcers on lungs: **Calc,** Carb-v, *Lyc,* **Phos,** Puls, Sep, **Sil,** *Sulf, Tub.*

Warm sense: **Sulf.**

Water: Sense of: Hot, in: **Acon,** *Hep*; boiling, poured into: [**Acon**].

Weakness: Acon, **Ant-t,** *Ars*, *Calc*, **Carb-v,** *Hep*, Iod, Nat-s, *Phos*, Rhus, **Seneg,** *Sil*, *Sulf*; from loud talking. Calc, **Sulf;** on waking: [**Carb-v**].

SLEEP

Comatose: Acon, **Ant-t,** *Ars*, **Bell,** *Bry*, *Lyc*, Merc, *Phos*, *Puls*, *Rhus*, Sep, *Sulf*.

Deep: Ant-t, *Ars*, **Bell,** *Bry*, *Calc*, **Carb-v,** *Chel*, *Hep*, *Lyc*, Merc, *Phos*, **Puls,** *Rhus*, *Seneg*, *Sulf*.

Disturbed: Acon, *Ars*, Bell, Merc, Puls, Sep, **Sulf.**

Dreams: Accidents: **Ars,** Bell, Iod, Lyc, Nat-s, Puls, Sulf; **anxious: Acon,** Ant-t, **Ars,** *Bell*, *Bry*, **Calc,** *Carb-v*, Chel, *Ferr-p*, *Hep*, *Iod*, Ipec, Lob, **Lyc,** *Merc*, *Nat-s*, **Phos, Puls, Rhus,** Sang, *Sep*, **Sil, Sulf; business:** Bell, *Bry*, Calc, Carb-v, *Chel*, Hep, *Lyc*, Merc, Phos, *Puls*, **Rhus,** Sang, *Sil*; **busy:** Bell, **Bry,** Lyc, Phos, Sang, Sep; **confused:** *Acon*, Ant-t, *Bry*, *Calc*, *Chel*, Ferr-p, Iod, *Lyc*, Phos, **Puls,** *Sep*, Sil, *Sulf*; of the **dead: Ars,** Bry, *Calc*, Iod, Lyc, *Phos*, Sil, *Sulf*; **difficulties:** Ant-t, **Ars,** *Phos*, Rhus; **events,** previous: *Acon*, *Ant-t*, *Bry*, Chel, Phos, *Rhus*, Sang, Sep, **Sil,** Sulf, of previous day: *Acon*, **Bry,** Chel, Lyc, Merc, *Puls*, Rhus, Sep, Sil, long past: **Sil;** of **falling:** Acon, **Bell,** Calc, Chel, Ferr-p, Hep, *Merc*, Nat-s, *Puls*, Sang, Sep, *Sulf*, **fire:** Ant-t, *Ars*, *Bell*, Calc, Carb-v, **Hep,** Merc, Nat-s, *Phos*, *Rhus*, Sil, *Sulf*; **frightful:** Acon, **Ars,** *Bell*, *Bry*, **Calc, Carb-v,** *Chel*, Hep, Ipec, **Lyc,** *Merc*, *Nat-s*, *Phos*, **Puls,** Rhus, Sang, Sep, **Sil,** *Sulf*, Verat-v; **misfortune:** *Ars*, *Bell*, **Lyc,** *Merc*, *Phos*, **Puls,** Rhus, *Sulf*; **nightmare:** *Acon*, Ant-t, Ars, Bell, *Bry*, *Calc*, Chel, Ferr-p, Hep, *Iod*, Lyc, Merc, Phos, Puls, Rhus, *Sil*, **Sulf,** lying on back: **Sulf;** roaming over **fields:** [**Rhus**]; **unpleasant:** Ant-t, Bry, Calc, Iod, Merc, Sang, Sep, **Sulf; vexatious:** *Ars*, *Bry*, Calc, Hep, Lyc, Nat-s, Phos, *Rhus*, Sep, Sil, **Sulf; vivid:** *Acon*, Ars, *Bell*, *Bry*, *Calc*, **Carb-v,** *Chel*, Ferr-p, *Iod*, Ipec, **Lyc,** *Merc*, **Phos,** *Puls*, **Rhus,** *Sep*, **Sil, Sulf,** Verat-v.

Falling asleep d. least mental exertion: **Ars,** Nat-s.

Sweat, d.: *Ars*, Bell, Chel, Lob, Phos, *Puls*, **Rhus.**

Position: Arms over head: Calc, **Puls,** Sulf, arms on abdomen: **Puls;** on back: Acon, Ant-t, Ars, **Bry,** *Calc*, Hep, *Lyc*, *Phos*, **Puls, Rhus,** *Sulf;* on r. side: **Phos,** on l. side impossible: Lyc, **Phos.**

Restless: Acon, *Ant-t*, **Ars, Bell,** *Bry*, *Calc*, *Carb-v*, *Chel*, Ferr-p, *Hep*, Iod, Ipec, **Lyc,** Merc, *Nat-s*, Phos, **Puls, Rhus,** Sang, Seneg, *Sep*, **Sil, Sulf; midnight,** a.: Bry, Lyc, **Rhus,** Sep, Sulf, 3 a. m.: **Ars,** Sulf.

Semi-conscious: Bell, Bry, Calc.

Sleepiness: *Acon*, **Ant-t, Ars, Bell,** *Bry*, *Calc*, **Carb-v, Chel,** *Ferr-p*, *Hep*, Iod, Ipec, Lob, *Lyc*, *Merc*, Nat-s, **Phos, Puls,** *Rhus*, Sang, Seneg, *Sep*, *Sil*, **Sulf,** Tub, Verat-v; **morning: Calc,** Hep, Lyc, *Merc*, *Nat-s*, *Phos*, *Puls*, Rhus, **Sep,** *Sil*, **Sulf; afternoon:** *Acon*, *Ars*, Bry, Carb-v, Chel, Lyc, Nat-s, Phos, *Puls*, **Rhus,** Sep, Sil, **Sulf; evening:** *Ant-t*, *Ars*, Bell, **Calc,** *Carb-v*, Chel, Ferr-p, *Hep*, Iod, Lyc, *Phos*, **Puls,** Rhus, Seneg, *Sep*, *Sil*, *Sulf*; **cough,** d.: **Ant-t,** *Ipec*; **dinner,** a.: Acon, Ant-t, Calc, *Carb-v*, Chel, **Lyc,** Nat-s, *Phos*, *Rhus*, Sil, Sulf; **eating,** a.: Acon, Bry, **Calc,** *Carb-v*, Chel, *Lyc*, *Phos*, *Rhus*, *Sil*, *Sulf*; **heat,** d.: Calc, Chel, Hep, *Lyc*, *Phos*, *Puls*, Rhus, Verat-v; mental **exertion: Ars,** Nat-s; overpowering afternoon: **Puls; supper,** a.: **Calc,** Carb-v; **vomiting,** a.: Bell, **Ipec.**

Sleeplessness: *Acon*, Ant-t, **Ars, Bell, Bry, Calc,** *Carb-v*, Ferr-p, **Hep,** *Iod*, *Ipec*, *Lyc*, **Merc,** *Nat-s*, **Phos, Puls, Rhus,** Sang, **Sep, Sil, Sulf; evening:** Bry, Calc, Lyc, Merc, *Phos*, **Puls,** *Rhus*, Sang, **Sulf,** heat: Calc, **Puls,** Rhus; **midnight:** b.: Acon, Ant-t, **Ars,** *Bell*, **Bry, Calc, Carb-v,** Chel, Ferr-p, *Hep*, Ipec, **Lyc, Merc, Phos, Puls, Rhus,** Seneg, **Sep, Sil, Sulf, a.:** *Acon*, **Ars,** Bell, Bry, **Hep,** *Iod*, Lyc, Puls, *Rhus*, *Sep*, **Sil,** a. **3 a. m.:** *Ars*, *Calc*, Rhus, **Sep, Sulf, a. 4 a. m.:** Phos, Sep, **Sulf,** a. **5 a. m.: Sulf; anxiety,** from: **Ars,** Bell, Bry, Merc, Rhus, Sulf; a. mental **exertion: Ars,** *Lyc*; from **shocks: Ars,** *Bell*, Ipec, *Phos*; though **sleepy:** *Acon*, Ars,

Bell, *Bry*, *Calc*, Carb-v, **Chel,** Ferr-p, *Hep*, Lyc, *Merc*, **Phos, Puls,** *Rhus*, **Sep,** *Sil*, *Sulf*; **thoughts,** activity of mind: Ant-t, **Ars,** Bell, *Bry*, **Calc, Hep,** *Lyc*, **Puls,** *Sep*, *Sil*, *Sulf*, *Tub*, same ideas always repeated: *Calc*, **Puls; twitching** of limbs: **Ars,** Bell, Calc, **Puls,** Rhus, Sep; a. **waking: Ars,** Bell, Calc, Carb-v, Ferr-p, Lyc, *Merc*, *Phos*, Puls, Rhus, *Sep*, **Sil,** *Sulf*; from **weariness:** [**Ars**].

Unrefreshing: Acon, Ant-t, *Ars*, *Bell*, Bry, Calc, Carb-v, *Chel*, Hep, *Lyc*, **Phos,** *Puls*, *Sep*, *Sil*, Sulf.

Waking: 3 a. m.: Ars, Sep, **Sulf; 5 a. m.:** urging to stool: **Sulf;** from **cold** limbs: [**Carb-v**]; from **cough** Ars, Calc, *Hep*, **Puls,** Rhus, Sep, Sil, **Sulf;** from **dreams:** *Bell*, Bry, *Hep*, Lyc, *Merc*, Phos, Puls, Sil, **Sulf; frequent:** *Acon*, Ant-t, *Ars*, *Bell*, *Bry*, **Calc,** *Carb-v*, Chel, **Hep,** Ipec, *Lyc*, *Merc*, Nat-s, **Phos, Puls,** *Rhus*, Sang, Seneg, **Sep,** *Sil*, **Sulf**; a. **midnight:** Sep, Sil, **Sulf;** as from **fright:** *Bell*, Chel, **Lyc,** Merc, *Puls*, Sang, *Sep*, **Sulf;** from **heat:** Ars, Calc, **Phos,** Sep, Sil, Sulf; from **hunger: Lyc.**

Yawning: *Acon*, *Ant-t*, **Ars,** Bell, *Bry*, *Calc*, Carb-v, **Chel,** Hep, Iod, Ipec, Lob, *Lyc*, Merc, Nat-s, *Phos*, *Puls*, **Rhus,** Sang, Seneg, *Sep*, *Sil*, Sulf; a. **cough: Ant-t,** *Ipec*; **frequent:** *Acon*, Ant-t, Bry, **Chel,** *Lyc*, Merc, Nat-s, Rhus, Sulf; b. **menses: Puls;** not **sleepy:** Acon, Ant-t, Bry, Hep, Phos, **Rhus,** *Sep*, Sulf; **spasmodic:** Acon, Ant-t, Bry, Calc, *Hep*, **Rhus,** Sep, Sulf.

CHILL

Morning: Acon, *Ars*, Bell, **Bry,** *Calc*, Carb-v, *Hep*, *Lyc*, *Merc*, Nat-s, *Phos*, **Sep,** Sil, *Sulf*; in bed: Lyc, **Merc,** Sulf.

Forenoon: Ant-t, **Ars, Calc,** *Lyc*, Phos, Sil, **Sulf.**

Noon: *Ars*, Bry, Chel, **Lob, Lyc,** Merc, Phos, **Puls,** Sil, *Sulf*, Tub.

Afternoon: Acon, Ant-t, **Ars,** *Bry*, *Chel*, Ferr-p, Ipec, **Lyc,** Phos, **Puls,** *Rhus*, *Sil*, *Sulf*; following heat: **Puls.**

Evening: Ant-t, Ars, **Bell, Bry,** *Calc, Carb-v, Chel,* **Hep, Lyc, Merc,** Nat-s, **Phos, Puls, Rhus, Sep,** Sil, **Sulf;** a. **lying** down: Acon, Bry, Lyc, Merc, Phos, **Puls;** d. **pain:** Puls; **7 p. m.** < by eating and drinking: [**Rhus**].

Night: Acon, *Ars, Bell,* Bry, Carb-v, Chel, Ferr-p, **Hep,** Iod, Ipec, Lyc, **Merc, Phos,** Puls, Rhus, Sep, Sil, **Sulf.**

Midnight: B.. *Phos,* **Puls,** Sulf; **a.: Ars,** *Hep,* Merc, Sil, Sulf.

Air, least draft: Bell, Bry, **Calc,** Hep, *Merc,* Sil, Sulf.

Anger, a.: Acon, Ars, **Bry.**

Anticipating: Ant-t, **Ars,** Bell, **Bry,** Sep.

Ascending: *Acon,* Ars, Calc, *Phos, Puls, Sep,* **Sulf.**

Bed, in: Acon, Ant-t, *Ars, Bell, Bry,* Calc, Carb-v, **Chel, Hep,** Iod, Ipec, **Lyc, Merc,** *Nat-s, Phos,* **Puls,** Rhus, Sang, Sep, **Sil, Sulf;** >: Bry, Puls, *Rhus,* Sulf; putting **hands** out of: **Hep,** Phos, **Rhus,** *Sil;* **rising** from: <: **Calc, Merc,** *Phos, Rhus, Sil,* >: Ant-t, Ars, Bell, **Iod,** *Lyc,* Merc, *Puls,* Rhus, *Sep,* Sulf; **turning** over in: Acon, *Bry,* Hep, Lyc, **Puls,** Sil, Sulf.

Beginning in: Finger tips: **Bry,** Puls, and toes: **Bry, Sep,** *Sulf;* lips: [**Bry**].

Chilliness lasting all day: **Sil; evening:** *Acon,* Bell, Bry, *Calc,* Carb-v, Hep, Lyc, Merc, *Nat-s,* Phos, **Puls,** *Rhus,* Sep, Sulf; b. **menses:** *Calc,* **Lyc, Puls,** *Sep,* **Sil, d.:** Bell, *Bry,* Calc, Ipec, *Phos,* **Puls, Sep, Sil, Sulf;** d. **sweat:** Acon, Ars, Bry, *Calc,* Phos, Puls, Sang, Sulf, **Tub.**

Disordered stomach: **Ipec,** *Puls.*

Drinking: <: Ant-t, **Ars,** Bry, **Calc,** *Chel,* Hep, *Lob,* Lyc, Puls, *Rhus,* Sep, Sil, Sulf; < the chill and causes vomiting: **Ars.**

Eating: A.: **Ars, Bell,** *Bry, Calc, Carb-v, Ipec, Lyc,* Phos, Puls, *Rhus,* Sep, Sil, *Sulf;* >: *Ars,* Chel, **Iod,** *Phos,* Rhus; **warm** things: <: *Bell,* Bry, **Puls; indiscrete: Ipec, Puls.**

Exposure: A.: *Acon*, *Ars*, *Bry*, **Calc**, Carb-v, *Hep*, *Nat-s*, **Rhus**, Sep; d. **rain:** Bell, *Calc*, **Nat-s, Rhus; swamps: Nat-s,** tropical countries: *Bry*, **Nat-s; wet,** to: Acon, Bell, *Bry*, *Calc*, *Nat-s*, **Rhus**, Sep, while overheated: Acon, *Calc*, **Rhus**, Sep, Sil; working in clay: [**Calc**,] in water: **Calc**, *Rhus*.

External: Acon, *Ant-t*, **Ars**, Bell, Bry, Calc, Chel, Iod, *Ipec*, *Merc*, Nat-s, *Phos*, Rhus, Sil, *Sulf*, *Verat-v*; in spots: Ars, Bell, Bry, Hep, Lyc, Merc, **Puls**, Rhus, **Sep**, *Sil*.

Heated: Overheated: Acon, Ant-t, Bell, *Bry*, **Carb-v**, *Nat-s*, Phos. **Puls**, Rhus, Sep, **Sil**.

Icy coldness of body: Ant-t, **Ars**, *Bry*, *Calc*, **Carb-v**, Nat-s, *Sep*, **Sil**; of skin of whole body, with cold breath: **Carb-v**.

Internal: *Acon*, **Ars**, *Bell*, *Bry*, **Calc**, Carb-v, *Chel*, **Hep**, Iod, *Ipec*, Lyc, **Merc**, *Nat-s*, **Phos, Puls**, *Rhus*, *Sep*, *Sil*, **Sulf; coldness** in bloodvessels: **Acon**, Ant-t, **Ars**, Lyc, **Rhus**.

Menses: B.: *Calc*, **Lyc, Puls**, Sep, **Sil**, Sulf; **d.:** *Bell*, Bry, *Calc*, Ipec, Lyc, *Nat-s*, *Phos*, **Puls, Sep, Sil, Sulf**.

Motion: *Acon*, *Ant-t*, Ars, *Bell*, **Bry**, *Hep*, Iod, Merc, **Rhus**, Sang, **Sep, Sil**, Sulf; >: *Acon*, Bell, Merc, **Puls**, Rhus, Sep, Sil; **a.: Ars**, Phos, **Puls, Rhus**, Sep.

Pain, d.: *Ars*, Bry, Hep, Lyc, **Puls**, *Rhus*, **Sep**, Sil, Sulf.

Sweat: With: *Ars*, Calc, Lyc, **Puls**, *Rhus*, Sang, Sulf; a. **chill:** Ars, Bry, *Carb-v*, **Lyc**, Phos, Puls, Rhus, *Sep*, Sulf.

Predominating: *Ant-t*, Ars, **Bry**, Carb-v, Hep, *Lyc*, Merc, Phos, *Puls*, Rhus, Sep, Sulf; **noon: Sulf; afternoon: Ars, Lyc, Puls**, *Rhus*; **evening:** *Hep*, *Phos*, **Puls, Rhus**, *Sulf*.

Shaking: Acon, *Ant-t*, **Ars**, *Bell*, *Bry*, *Calc*, *Carb-v*, **Chel**, Ferr-p, **Hep**, *Iod*, *Ipec*, *Lob*, **Lyc**, *Merc*, *Nat-s*,

Phos, Puls, Rhus, Sang, **Sep,** *Sil,* **Sulf; forenoon: Phos,** Puls; **afternoon: Ars,** Chel, Ipec, **Phos,** *Rhus,* Sulf; **evening: Ars,** *Carb-v,* **Chel,** *Hep,* **Lyc,** *Merc,* Nat-s, *Phos, Sep, Sil,* Sulf; putting **hands** out of bed: **Hep,** Phos, **Rhus; heat** of head: **Bell,** Bry; heat without thirst: **Sep,** *Sulf.*

Sides: One: Ant-t, Bell, **Bry, Carb-v,** *Chel,* **Lyc,** *Phos,* **Puls, Rhus,** *Sep,* **Sil,** *Sulf;* **l.: Carb-v, Lyc,** *Rhus,* Sulf; **r.: Bry, Chel,** *Lyc, Phos,* Puls, **Rhus.**

Single parts: Ars, Bell, Bry, *Calc,* Hep, Lyc, **Puls,** Rhus, **Sep,** Sil.

Sleep:> a.: Ars, Bry, Calc, **Phos,** Rhus, Sep.

Time: 1 a. m.: Ars, Puls, Sil; 2 a. m.: Ars, Hep, Puls, Rhus, Sil; 12 m. to 2 p. m.: Ars, Sulf; 1 p. m.: Ars, Chel, Ferr-p, Merc, Phos, Puls, Sil, Sulf, to 2 p. m..: Ars, Merc, Puls; 2 p. m.: Ars, Calc, Chel, Lob, Puls, Sang, Sil, Sulf; 3 p. m.: Ant-t, Ars, Bell, Calc, Chel, Lyc, Puls, Sil; 4 p. m.; Ars, Chel, Hep, Ipec, Lyc, Nat-s, Puls, Sep, Sil, Sulf, to 8 p. m.: Hep, Lyc, Nat-s; 5 p. m.: Ars, Chel, Hep, Ipec, Lyc, Phos, Rhus, Sep, Sil, Sulf, Tub; 6 p. m.: Ant-t, Ars, Bell, Chel, Hep, Lyc, Nat-s, Phos, Puls, Rhus, Sep, Sil, Sulf, til 5 a. m.: Hep; 7. p. m.: Ars, Calc, Chel, Hep, Lyc, Nat-s, Phos, Puls, Rhus, Sil, Sulf, Tub.

Touch:<: **Acon,** Bell, Hep, *Lyc,* Phos, Puls, Sep, Sulf.

Trembling: Shivering: Acon, **Ant-t,** Ars, Bell, Bry, Calc, Merc, Phos, *Puls,* Rhus, **Sil,** Sulf.

Uncovering: Undressing, on: *Acon, Ars, Bell, Calc,* **Hep,** *Merc, Phos, Puls,* **Rhus,** *Sep,* **Sil.**

Warm: Room: *Acon,* Bry, **Ipec,** Merc, Puls, *Sep,*>: **Ars,** Bell, Carb-v, **Chel,** *Hep,* Merc, *Rhus, Sep,* Sil, Sulf; does not> nor does stove: *Acon,* Ars, Bell, **Bry,** Calc, Hep, Iod, **Ipec,** Lyc, *Merc, Phos,* **Puls,** *Sep, Sil,* Sulf; **weather:** *Ars, Bell, Bry,* Calc, Carb-v, *Ipec,* Puls, **Sulf.**

Warmth: Ext.:>: **Ars, Bell,** Chel, *Hep,* **Rhus,** Sep, Sil, Sulf.

Water: Cold, dashed over one, as if: Ant-t, Ars, Bry, *Chel*, Lyc, Merc, *Phos*, *Puls*, **Rhus,** poured over him, as if: *Ant-t*, Ars, **Merc,** *Rhus*; **wetting,** on: Acon, Bell, *Bry*, *Calc*, *Nat-s*, **Rhus,** *Sep*, Sil, **working** in, from: **Calc,** *Rhus*.

FEVER

Morning, bed, in: Ars, **Puls,** Sulf.

10 a. m. as if dashed with, or as of hot water running through bloodvessels: [**Rhus**].

Afternoon: Acon, Ant-t, Ars, **Bell,** *Bry*, Calc, *Chel*, Hep, Iod, Ipec, *Lyc*, **Phos, Puls,** Rhus, *Sang*, *Sep*, *Sil*, Sulf; alt. with **chill: Calc;** a. lying down: Bry, Chel, **Puls,** Sulf; **2 p. m.: Puls,** Rhus, Sang, followed by chill at 4 p. m.: [**Puls**].

Evening: Acon, Ant-t, *Ars*, **Bell,** Bry, *Calc*, *Carb-v*, *Chel*, *Hep*, Ipec, **Lyc,** *Merc*, **Phos, Puls, Rhus,** *Sep*, **Sil,** *Sulf*; in **bed** a. lying down: *Acon*, **Bry,** Chel; on entering **room: Puls,** Sulf, **6 to 8 p. m.: Lyc.**

Night: *Acon*, Ant-t, *Ars*, **Bell, Bry,** *Calc*, *Carb-v*, *Hep*, *Lyc*, **Merc,** *Nat-s*, **Phos, Puls, Rhus,** *Sep*, **Sil, Sulf,** *Tub*; with **chilliness:** Acon, *Ars*, Carb-v, *Rhus*, *Sil*, **Sulf,** Tub; dry, burning, **heat: Acon, Ars, Bell, Bry,** Calc, Carb-v, Chel, Hep, Lyc, **Phos,** *Puls*, **Rhus,** *Tub*, without **thirst: Ars,** with **anxiety:** Acon, **Ars,** Bry, Rhus; with **sweat: Bell,** Bry, Calc, **Merc, Phos, Puls, Rhus,** *Sep*, **Sulf;** on **waking:** Carb-v. **Sulf; 9 p. m.: Bry,** Lyc.

Midnight: Ars, Lyc, *Rhus*, Sep, Sulf; **b.:** Acon, Ars, **Bry,** *Carb-v*, Lyc, Phos, Puls, Sep; **a.: Ars,** *Lyc*, Merc, Phos, Sulf.

Alt. with chills: Acon, *Ant-t*, **Ars, Bell, Bry, Calc,** Chel, **Hep,** *Iod*, *Ipec*, Lob, *Lyc*, **Merc,** Nat-s, *Phos*, Puls, **Rhus,** *Sang*, *Sep*, *Sil*, Sulf; **night: Acon,** Ipec, *Merc*, Phos, Sep, Sulf.

Anger, from: Acon, **Sep.**

Ascending: *Acon*, Ant-t, Bell, Lyc, **Phos, Sep, Sulf.**

Bed, in: *Acon*, Ant-t, *Bry*, *Calc*, *Carb-v*, Chel, Hep, **Merc,** Phos, **Puls,** *Rhus*, Sil, *Sulf.*

Burning heat: **Acon,** Ant-t, **Ars, Bell,** *Bry*, *Carb-v*, Chel, *Hep*, Ipec, *Lyc*, Merc, **Phos, Puls,** *Rhus*, Sulf, **Tub; afternoon:** Ars, **Bell,** *Bry*, *Hep*, Lyc, **Phos,** *Puls*, Rhus, Sulf, **4 p. m.** lasting several hours: [**Lyc**]; **evening:** *Acon*, *Ars*, **Bell,** *Bry*, *Carb-v*, Hep, Ipec, **Lyc, Phos, Puls, Rhus,** Sulf; **night: Acon, Ars, Bell,** *Bry*, *Carb-v*, *Hep*, Lyc, Merc, **Phos, Puls,** *Rhus*, Sulf, in **bed,** intolerable burning: [**Puls**]; **midnight: Ars,** Lyc, *Rhus*, Sulf, **b.:** Ars, **Bry,** Puls, Sep, **a.: Ars,** Lyc, Merc, *Phos*, Sulf; alt. with **chilliness:** [**Bell**]; **heat** outside, cold inside: [**Ars**]; **int.** mostly, blood seems to burn in veins: **Ars,** *Bry*, **Rhus;** spreading from **hands** over whole body: [**Chel**]; with **thirst:** for cold drinks: *Acon*, **Phos,** unquenchable: **Ars,** Bell, Hep, **Phos;** int. and ext., body burning hot: [**Bell**].

Chill absent: Acon, **Ars, Bell, Bry,** *Calc*, Carb-v, *Ferr-p*, Hep, *Ipec*, *Lyc*, Puls, **Rhus,** Sulf; **afternoon: Ars, Bell,** *Bry*, Calc, Ipec, Lyc, Puls, Rhus, *Sang*, *Sil*, Sulf, 1 to 2 p. m.: [**Ars**], 2 p. m.: [**Puls**], 4 p. m.: Ars, Hep, *Ipec*, **Lyc; evening:** Acon, Ant-t, Ars, **Bell, Bry,** Calc, Carb-v, Ferr-p, Hep, Ipec, Lyc, **Puls, Rhus,** Sulf; **night:** Acon, Ant-t, **Ars, Bell, Bry,** *Calc*, *Carb-v*, Hep, Ipec, Lyc, *Phos*, *Puls*, **Rhus,** Sulf; **midnight: Ars,** Sulf, **b.:** Acon, Ars, **Bry,** *Carb-v*, Lyc, Puls, **a.: Ars,** Lyc, Sulf, 12 to 2 a. m.: [**Ars**], 12 to 3 a. m.: **Ars,** 1 to 2 a. m.: [**Ars**], 2 a. m.: **Ars.**

Chill, with **Acon, Ars, Bell,** *Bry*, **Calc,** Carb-v, Chel, Iod, Ipec, Lyc, *Merc*, *Nat-s*, Phos, *Puls*, **Rhus,** *Sang*, *Sep*, Sil, **Sulf.**

Chilliness, with: Acon, *Ars*, *Bell*, **Calc,** Carb-v, Hep, *Merc*, Phos, **Puls,** *Sep*, Sil, *Sulf*, *Tub*, from putting hands out of bed: *Hep*, **Tub.**

Continued: *Ant-t*, **Bry,** *Carb-v*, Chel, *Lyc*, **Phos,** *Rhus*, *Sulf.*

Dry heat: **Acon,** Ant-t, **Ars, Bell, Bry,** *Calc,* Carb-v, Chel, *Ferr-p,* Hep, *Iod,* Ipec, *Lyc, Merc,* Nat-s, **Phos,** *Puls, Rhus,* Sep, Sil, *Sulf;* **evening:** Ars, Bell, Carb-v, **Puls,** distended veins and burning hands that seek cool places: [**Puls**]; **night: Acon,** Ant-t, **Ars, Bell,** *Bry,* Calc, Carb-v, Chel, Hep, Lyc, **Phos,** *Puls,* **Rhus,** with delirium: **Ars, Bell,** *Bry, Lyc, Phos,* **Rhus.**

Eating, a.: Bell, *Bry,* Calc, Lyc, **Phos,** *Sep,* Sil, Sulf.

Ext. heat: **Acon,** *Ant-t,* **Ars, Bell, Bry,** *Calc, Carb-v,* Chel, Hep, Iod, Ipec, *Lyc, Merc, Phos,* **Puls, Rhus,** Sep, **Sil,** *Sulf,* with **chilliness:** *Acon,* **Ars,** *Bell, Bry,* **Calc,** Hep, *Lyc,* Merc, *Phos,* **Sep,** *Sil, Sulf;* desire to be **fanned** in place of thirst: [**Carb-v**].

Heat absent: *Hep, Lyc,* Rhus, **Sulf.**

Hectic fever: **Ars,** Bry, *Calc, Carb-v,* Ferr-p, Hep, **Iod,** Ipec, **Lyc,** *Merc,* **Phos,** *Puls,* **Sang, Sep, Sil,** *Sulf,* **Tub.**

Intense heat: **Acon,** Ant-t, **Ars, Bell,** *Bry,* Chel, Hep, *Lyc,* Nat-s, *Phos,* **Puls, Rhus,** Sang, *Sil, Tub;* with delirium: Ant, **Ars, Bell,** *Bry,* Carb-v, Hep, Iod, **Puls.**

Int. heat: **Acon, Ars, Bell, Bry,** *Calc, Carb-v,* Chel, *Ferr-p, Iod,* Ipec, *Lyc,* **Merc, Phos,** *Puls,* **Rhus,** *Sep, Sil,* **Sulf;** burning in bloodvessels: **Ars,** *Bry, Calc,* **Rhus,** *Sulf;* ext. **chill: Acon, Ars,** *Bell,* Bry, *Calc, Chel, Iod, Ipec, Phos, Puls, Rhus,* Sang, *Sil,* Sulf.

Irregular stages: **Ars, Bry,** *Ipec, Sep.*

Irritative fever: Acon, **Ars,** Bell, *Bry, Carb-v, Lyc,* Merc, *Puls, Rhus,* Sulf; **slow: Ars,** *Bry, Lyc, Phos,* Sil, Sulf.

Menses: d.: *Acon, Bell,* Bry, *Calc,* Merc, *Phos,* **Sep,** *Sulf.*

Motion brings on chilliness: Ant-t, *Merc,* **Rhus;** desires quiet in all stages: **Bry.**

Paroxysms: < in severity: Ars, *Bry,* **Puls;** irregular: **Ars,** Carb-v, *Ipec,* **Puls, Sep,** long chill, little heat, no thirst: [**Puls**], one stage wanting: **Ars,** Lyc, short chill, long heat, no thirst: [**Ipec**].

Paroxysmal fever: *Bry, Calc,* Hep, Lyc, *Merc;* night: **Merc.**

Sweat: Absent: Acon, **Ars, Bell, Bry,** Calc, Iod, *Ipec, Lyc, Phos,* Puls, *Rhus,* Sang, Sil, *Sulf,* Tub; with **heat:** Ant-t, *Bell,* Bry, *Calc,* Carb-v, Chel, Hep, *Ipec, Merc, Nat-s,* **Phos, Puls,** *Rhus, Sep,* **Sulf, Tub.**

Relapsing: Ars, **Calc, Sulf,** *Tub.*

Remittent: Acon, *Ant-t,* **Ars, Bell, Bry,** *Ipec, Lyc,* **Merc,** *Nat-s,* Phos, Puls, Rhus, Sep, *Sulf,* **afternoon: Ars, Bell,** *Bry, Lyc;* **evening:** *Acon,* **Bell,** *Bry,* **Lyc,** Merc, *Phos,* Puls, **Rhus,** *Sulf;* **night:** Ant-t, **Ars,** Lyc, **Merc,** *Phos, Puls,* **Rhus,** *Sulf;* **infants: Acon,** Ars, **Bell,** *Bry, Ipec,* Sulf; prone to become typhoid: Ant-t, **Ars, Bry,** Phos, **Rhus,** Tub.

Shivering, with: Acon, Ant-t, *Bell,* Bry, *Calc,* Carb-v, *Hep,* Merc, Puls, *Rhus,* Sep, **Sulf;** uncovering, from: *Calc, Rhus,* **Tub.**

Side: One: *Bell,* **Bry,** Carb-v, Chel, **Lyc,** *Phos,* **Puls,** *Rhus, Sulf;* **r.:** *Bell, Bry,* Carb-v, **Phos,** *Puls,* Tub; **l.:** Bell, **Lyc,** Merc, **Rhus,** *Sulf,* with coldness of r.: **Rhus;** one cheek red and hot, the other pale and cold: [**Acon**].

Sleep, fever comes on a.: Ars, *Bell,* Calc, Ferr-p, Hep, Ipec, Lyc, Merc, *Phos,* Puls, *Sep, Sil,* **Sulf.**

Succession of stages: Chill then heat: **Acon,** *Ant-t,* Ars, *Bell,* Bry, Calc, *Carb-v, Hep,* **Iod, Ipec, Lyc,** Merc, *Nat-s, Phos,* **Puls, Rhus, Sang,** Seneg, Sep, Sil, **Sulf;** chill, then heat, then sweat: **Ars,** Bell, *Bry,* Carb-v, Hep, **Ipec,** Lyc, *Nat-s,* **Puls,** *Rhus,* Sep, *Sulf;* chill then heat with sweat: *Acon,* Ant-t, **Bell,** Bry, Carb-v, *Hep,* Phos, *Puls,* **Rhus,** Sulf; chill then sweat without intervening heat: *Bry,* Carb-v, Chel, **Lyc,** Merc, Nat-s, Phos, *Rhus,* Sep; heat then chill: *Bell, Bry,* **Calc,** Lyc, Merc, *Phos,*

Puls, Sep, *Sulf*, *Tub*; heat then sweat: Ant-t, **Ars,** Bell, Bry, Calc, *Carb-v*, Hep, *Ipec*, Lob, Lyc, Puls, **Rhus,** *Sil*, Sulf.

Uncovering: Aversion to: Acon, Ars, **Bell,** *Calc*, *Hep*, *Merc*, Phos, **Puls, Rhus,** *Sil*, **Tub; desires: Acon,** *Ars*, Bry, Calc, *Hep*, Iod, Lyc, *Phos*, **Puls,** Rhus, *Sulf*; causes **chilliness:** Acon, *Bell*, *Calc*, **Rhus,** *Sep*, **Tub,** in any stage of paroxysm: Ars, *Hep*, **Rhus.**

Vexation causes heat: Acon, Phos, **Sep.**

Warm covering:<: Acon, Calc, Lyc, **Puls,** Rhus, Sulf; room:< · *Bry*, *Ipec*, *Lyc*, **Puls,** *Sulf*.

Warmth:<: Bry, **Puls.**

Washing:>: Puls.

PERSPIRATION

Daytime: *Ant-t*, Bell, Bry, **Calc,** *Ferr-p*, *Hep*, **Lyc,** *Merc*, Puls, **Sep,** *Sil*, **Sulf;** night and, without>: **Hep;** with nausea and languor: [**Merc**].

Morning: Acon, *Ars*, Bell, *Bry*, **Calc, Carb-v,** *Chel*, Ferr-p, **Hep,** Iod, *Lyc*, **Merc, Phos,** *Puls*, *Rhus*, Sang, *Sep*, **Sil,** *Sulf*, in **bed: Calc,** Lyc, Phos; a. **heat:** Ars, **Puls;** d. **sleep:** Bell, *Chel*, **Puls;** a. **waking:** Ant-t, Bry, Carb-v, Chel, Phos, **Sep, Sulf.**

Evening: Bed, in: Ars, Calc, **Merc, Sulf;** lasting all night: Chel, **Hep, Puls.**

Night: Acon, Ant-t, **Ars,** Bell, Bry, *Calc*, **Carb-v,** *Ferr-p*, **Hep,** *Iod*, *Ipec*, Lob, *Lyc*, **Merc,** Nat-s, Phos, **Puls,** *Rhus*, **Sep, Sil, Sulf;** lasting all night without>: **Hep, Merc.** with loquacity: [**Puls**]; d. sleep: Ant-t, *Bell*, Chel, Phos, **Puls,** d. stupid slumber: [**Puls**].

Midnight: A. Acon, Ars, *Chel*, Lyc, Merc, Phos, Puls, *Sil*, Sulf, **Tub, 4 a. m.** d. sleep: **Chel.**

Affected parts, on: **Ant-t,** Ars, Bry, **Merc, Rhus,** *Sep*, Sil.

Air, cold: Ars, **Bry, Calc,** *Lyc,* Sep.

Anger, from: Acon, Bry, Lyc, **Sep.**

Anxiety, d.: **Ars,** Bry, **Calc,** *Carb-v, Merc, Phos, Puls, Rhus,* **Sep,** Sil, *Sulf;* night: **Ars,** *Carb-v.*

Bed: In: Ars, Bry, **Calc,** Iod, Lyc, *Merc,* Phos, *Rhus,* Sep, *Sulf;* > getting out of: Ars, Bell, *Calc,* Hep, Lyc, *Merc, Puls,* **Rhus,** *Sep,* Sulf.

Clammy: Acon, *Ant-t,* **Ars,** *Calc,* Carb-v, **Ferr-p,** *Hep,* Iod, **Lyc, Merc, Phos,** *Tub.*

Cold: *Acon,* **Ant-t, Ars,** Bell, *Bry, Calc,* **Carb-v, Hep,** Iod, **Ipec,** *Lob,* **Lyc,** *Merc, Phos, Puls,* Rhus, Sang, Seneg, **Sep,** Sil, *Sulf, Tub,* **Verat-v; night:** Iod, Lob, Rhus, **Sep;** while eating :[**Merc**]; least bodily or mental exertion: *Calc,* **Hep, Sep.**

Colliquative: Ant-t, *Ars, Carb-v, Lyc.*

Coughing, from: Acon, Ant-t, **Ars,** Bell, Bry, *Calc, Carb-v,* **Hep,** *Ipec,* Lyc, *Merc,* **Phos,** Puls, *Rhus,* Seneg, **Sep,** Sil, Sulf.

Covered parts: **Acon, Bell,** *Puls.*

Dyspnea, with: *Ant-t,* **Ars, Carb-v,** Lyc, Sil, Sulf.

Eating, d.: Ant-t, Ars, Bry, *Calc,* **Carb-v, Merc,** Phos, *Puls,* **Sep,** Sil;>: **Phos;** anxiety and cold sweat: [**Merc**]; **a.:** Ars, **Bry, Calc, Carb-v,** *Lyc,* **Phos, Sep,** Sil, **Sulf; warm** food: *Bry, Carb-v,* **Phos,** Puls, Sep.

Exertion, slight: Acon, *Ars,* Bell, *Bry,* **Calc,** Carb-v, *Chel,* Ferr-p, *Hep,* **Iod, Lyc,** *Merc,* **Nat-s, Phos, Rhus, Sep,** *Sil,* **Sulf; mental:** Bell, **Calc, Hep,** Lyc, Phos, **Sep,** Sil, *Sulf,* Tub.

Fever, a.: Ant-t, **Ars,** Bell, Bry, Calc, Carb-v, *Hep, Lyc, Nat-s, Phos, Puls, Rhus.*

Head, except: *Bell,* Merc, **Rhus,** *Sep.*

Hot: Acon, *Bell,* Bry, Calc, *Carb-v,* Chel, **Ipec,** Phos, Puls, **Sep,** Sil, *Sulf.*

Long lasting: *Ars,* **Hep.**

Lying, while: Ars, Chel, Hep, Lyc, Merc, Puls, **Rhus,** *Sep.*

Motion: Ant-t, *Ars,* Bell, **Bry, Calc,** Carb-v, **Hep,** Iod, Ipec, **Merc,** Phos, Puls, **Sep,** Sil, **Sulf;** >: *Ars,* **Merc,** *Puls,* **Rhus,** Sep, Sulf.

Odor: Fetid: **Hep,** Lyc, *Merc, Tub*; **offensive:** *Ars,* Bell, *Carb-v,* **Hep, Lyc, Merc,** *Phos,* **Puls,** *Rhus,* **Sep, Sil, Sulf,** night: Ars, Carb-v, **Merc,** Rhus; **putrid: Carb-v,** Rhus; **sour:** *Acon,* **Ars, Bry,** Calc, *Carb-v,* Chel, **Hep, Iod,** *Ipec,* **Lyc, Merc,** Puls, *Rhus,* **Sep, Sil, Sulf,** morning: *Bry, Carb-v, Iod,* Lyc, Rhus, **Sulf,** night: Ars, Bry, **Hep,** Iod, Lyc, *Sep, Sulf.*

Oily: Bry, Calc, **Merc;** night: Bry, **Merc.**

Pain from: Acon, *Ant-t,* Bell, *Bry,* Calc, *Chel, Hep,* Lyc, **Merc,** Rhus, **Sep,** *Sulf.*

Profuse: *Acon,* **Ant-t, Ars, Bell, Bry, Calc, Carb-v,** Chel, *Ferr-p,* **Hep,** Iod, *Ipec,* Lob, **Lyc, Merc,** *Phos, Puls, Rhus,* Sang, **Sep, Sil,** *Sulf,* **Tub,** Verat-v; **morning:** Acon, Ars, Bry, Carb-v, *Merc,* **Phos,** *Puls, Rhus,* Sep, **Sil,** a. waking: *Sep,* **Sulf; night:** *Ant-t, Ars, Bry, Carb-v,* Chel, *Ferr-p,* **Hep,** Iod, *Lob, Lyc,* **Merc, Phos, Sil, Sulf,** with sleeplessness: Iod, **Sulf;** on affected parts: [**Ant-t**]; **day** and **night** without>: **Hep,** *Merc*; on **waking:** *Sep,* **Sulf.**

Room, in: Acon, Bry, **Ipec,** *Phos,* **Puls,** Rhus, Sep, Sulf.

Sides: One: Acon, Bell, *Bry,* Lyc, Merc, *Phos,* **Puls,** Rhus, *Sulf*; **L.:** Phos, **Puls,** Rhus.

Single parts: *Acon,* Ars, Bell, *Bry,* **Calc,** Hep, Ipec, *Lyc,* Merc, **Puls,** Rhus. **Sep,** *Sil,* Sulf, *Tub*; **front** of body: *Calc,* Merc, **Phos.**

Sitting, while: **Ars,** *Calc,* Lyc, Phos, *Rhus,* Sep, Sulf.

Sleep: Beginning: **Ars,** *Calc,* Lyc, **Merc,** *Phos,* Puls, Rhus, *Sep,* Sil, **Sulf; d.:** *Ant-t, Ars,* **Bell,** Bry, Calc, Carb-v, **Chel,** *Ferr-p,* Hep, Lyc, *Merc, Phos,* **Puls, Rhus,** *Sep,* **Sil,** *Sulf,* Tub; **waking,** a.: *Ars,*

Bell, Bry, *Calc*, Carb-v, *Chel*, Hep, Lyc, *Merc*, *Phos*, **Sep,** Sil, **Sulf,** >: *Ars*, Bell, **Chel, Phos, Puls,** *Sep*, Sil, *Sulf.*

Stains linen: Ars, **Bell,** Merc; yellow: Ars, *Bell*, Bry, Ipec, **Merc,** Tub.

Stool: B.: *Acon*, Ant-t, *Bell*, Bry, Calc, **Merc,** Phos, Rhus; **d.:** Acon, Ars, Bell, Calc, Carb-v, Hep, Ipec, **Merc,** Rhus, Sep, *Sulf*; **a.: Acon,** Ars, Calc, Carb-v, *Merc*, Phos, Rhus, Sep, Sulf, warm, becomes cold and sticky: [**Merc**].

Suddenly, comes and goes: [**Bell**].

Suppression, from: *Acon*, *Ars*, **Bell, Bry, Calc,** *Carb-v*, Hep, *Lyc*, *Merc*, *Nat-s*, *Phos*, Puls, **Rhus,** Seneg, **Sep, Sil, Sulf.**

Symptoms, sweat<: *Acon*, Ant-t, **Ars,** Calc, *Ipec*, Lyc. **Merc,** Phos, Puls, **Rhus, Sep, Sulf;** >: *Acon*, *Ars*, Bell, **Bry,** *Hep*, Lyc, **Rhus; a.:**<: *Acon*, Ant-t, Ipec, *Merc*, Phos, *Puls*, **Sep,** Sil, *Sulf.*

Uncovering: Aversion to: Acon, Ars, *Calc*, Hep, **Rhus,** Sil, Tub; >: Acon, *Bell*, Calc, **Lyc,** *Puls*, Sulf.

Vexation, a.: Acon, Bry, Lyc, **Sep.**

Warmth causing uneasiness: **Calc,** *Puls*, **Sep,** *Sulf.*

Writing, while: *Hep*, **Sep,** *Sulf*, *Tub.*

GENERALS

Daytime: *Puls*, *Rhus*, *Sang*, **Sep, Sulf.**

Morning: *Acon*, *Ars*, Bell, **Bry, Calc, Carb-v, Chel,** *Ferr-p*, *Hep*, Iod, Ipec, Lyc, *Merc*, **Nat-s, Phos, Puls, Rhus,** *Sang*, *Seneg*, **Sep,** *Sil*, **Sulf,** *Verat-v*; **11** a. m.: Ars, Ipec, **Sulf.**

Forenoon: Ant-t, Ars, Bell, *Bry*, Calc, *Carb-v*, Chel, Ipec, Merc, Puls, *Rhus*, Seneg, **Sep,** *Sil*, **Sulf;**>: **Lyc.**

Noon, a. eating:>: **Chel.**

Afternoon: Acon, Ant-t, *Ars*, **Bell**, *Bry*, Calc, Carb-v, *Chel*, Ferr-p, Iod, Ipec, **Lyc**, *Merc*, *Phos*, **Puls**, **Rhus**, *Sang*, *Seneg*, **Sep**, **Sil**, *Sulf*; **3** p. m.: Ars, **Bell**, Sil, Sulf; **4** p. m.: Carb-v, Chel, **Lyc**, Nat-s, Puls, to 8 p. m.: **Lyc**, Sulf.

Evening: *Acon*, **Ant-t**, *Ars*, **Bell**, **Bry**, **Calc**, **Carb-v**, Chel, *Ferr-p*, *Hep*, *Iod*, *Ipec*, **Lyc**, **Merc**, **Phos**, **Puls**, *Rhus*, *Sang*, *Seneg*, **Sep**, **Sil**, **Sulf**; **twilight<:** *Ars*, *Calc*, *Phos*, **Puls**, Rhus; **9** p. m.: **Bry**, Sulf.

Night: **Acon**, *Ant-t*, **Ars**, *Bell*, *Bry*, **Calc**, *Carb-v*, Chel, *Ferr-p*, **Hep**, **Iod**, **Ipec**, *Lyc*, **Merc**, *Nat-s*, **Phos**, **Puls**, **Rhus**, Sang, Seneg, **Sep**, **Sil**, **Sulf**.

Midnight: B.: *Ant-t*, **Ars**, ~~*Bell*~~, *Bry*, **Carb-v**, Chel, *Hep*, **Lyc**, *Merc*, **Phos**, **Puls**, ~~*Rhus*~~, *Sep*, Sulf; **a.:** Acon, Ant-t, **Ars**, Bell, *Bry*, *Calc*, Carb-v, *Chel*, Ferr-p, Hep, Iod, *Merc*, Nat-s, **Phos**, *Puls*, **Rhus**, Seneg, Sep, **Sil**, *Sulf*, **>: [Lyc].**

Air: Draft<: Acon, *Ars*, **Bell**, Bry, **Calc**, *Hep*, *Lyc*, *Merc*, *Phos*, Puls, **Rhus**, *Sep*, **Sil**; **Open:** aversion to: *Bell*, *Bry*, **Calc**, Carb-v, Chel, *Hep*, Ipec, *Lyc*, *Merc*, Phos, *Rhus*, Seneg, *Sep*, **Sil**, **Sulf**, **desire** for: Acon, Ant-t, *Ars*, *Bry*, **Carb-v**, **Iod**, **Lyc**, *Nat-s*, Phos, **Puls**, Rhus, Seneg, Sep, **Sulf**.

Anemia: Acon, **Ars**, *Bell*, *Bry*, **Calc**, *Carb-v*, *Ferr-p*, Iod, Lyc, **Merc**, *Nat-s*, **Phos**, **Puls**, *Rhus*, *Sep*, Sil, **Sulf**.

Anxiety, general physical: Acon, *Ant-t*, **Ars**, *Bry*, *Calc*, Carb-v, *Chel*, *Ferr-p*, *Iod*, **Ipec**, Lob, *Lyc*, Merc, **Phos**, **Puls**, Rhus, Seneg, *Sep*, **Sulf**.

Bathing: Dread of: *Bell*, *Bry*, *Calc*, *Carb-v*, Lyc, Merc, Phos, *Puls*, **Rhus**, **Sep**, Sil, **Sulf**; **<:** Ant-t, *Bell*, Bry, **Calc**, *Carb-v*, *Lyc*, *Merc*, *Phos*, Puls, **Rhus**, **Sep**, Sil, **Sulf**; **>:** Acon, Ant-t, Ars, Bry, *Chel*, **Puls**, Sep; the **affected part>:** Ant-t, Ars, Bry, *Chel*, **Puls**, Sep; **cold<:** *Bell*, Phos, **Rhus**, *Sep*, **Tub.**

Breakfast, a.:<: Ars, Bell, *Bry*, *Calc*, Carb-v, Lyc, **Phos**, Puls, Rhus, *Sep*, Sil, *Sulf*.

Burns, a.: **Ars,** Calc, *Carb-v*, *Rhus*.

Change of: Position<: Acon, *Bry*, *Carb-v*, *Chel*, *Lyc*, *Phos*. **Puls,** Rhus, Sil,>: Ars, *Nat-s*, Puls, **Rhus; temperature<:** Acon, **Ars,** *Carb-v*, Lyc, Phos, *Puls*, Rhus, Sulf; **weather<:** *Ant-t*, Ars, *Bell*, *Bry*, *Calc*, *Chel*, Hep, Merc, **Phos,** *Puls*, **Rhus,** Sep, **Sil,** *Sulf*, **Tub,** cold to warm<: **Bry,** Carb-v, *Chel*, *Lyc*, *Nat-s*, *Puls*, **Sulf, Tub.**

Chlorotic subjects: **Ars, Bell, Calc,** *Carb-v*, Ferr-p, *Hep*, **Lyc,** Merc, **Phos, Puls, Sep, Sulf.**

Clothing: Intolerable: *Bry*, **Calc,** *Carb-v*, Hep, **Lyc,** *Nat-s*, *Puls*, *Sep*, Sulf; **loosening>:** *Bry*, **Calc,** *Carb-v*, Chel, *Hep*, **Lyc,** *Puls*, *Sep*, *Sulf*.

Cold: Air<: *Acon*, **Ars,** *Bell*, *Bry*, **Calc,** *Carb-v*, Ferr-p, **Hep,** *Ipec*, **Lyc,** *Merc*, *Phos*, *Puls*, **Rhus,** Seneg, **Sep, Sil,** *Sulf*; **becoming:** Acon, **Ars,** Bell, *Bry*, *Calc*, *Carb-v*, Ferr-p, **Hep, Lyc,** Merc, *Phos*, **Rhus, Sep, Sil,** *Sulf*,>: Acon, Ant-t, Bell, *Bry*, Carb-v, **Iod,** Ipec, **Lyc,** *Merc*, Phos, **Puls,** Seneg, *Sulf*, **a.<:** *Acon*, *Ant-t*, **Ars, Bell, Bry, Calc,** *Carb-v*, **Hep,** *Ipec*, *Lyc*, **Merc, Phos, Puls, Rhus, Sep. Sil,** *Sulf*, a **part** of the body<: *Bell*, **Hep,** Puls, **Rhus,** *Sep*, **Sil,** feet: Puls, **Sil,** hands out of bed: **Hep,** Phos, **Rhus,** *Sil*, head: **Bell,** Puls, **Sep, Sil;** dry **weather** <: **Acon,** *Ars*, Bell, *Bry*, Carb-v, **Hep,** *Ipec*, Sep, *Sil*, Sulf; entering a, **place:**<: **Ars,** Carb-v, *Hep*, Phos, *Puls*, *Rhus*, **Sep,** *Sil*, *Tub*; tendency to **take: Acon,** Ant-t, Ars, *Bell*, **Bry,** *Calc*, *Carb-v*, Ferr-p, **Hep,** Iod, Ipec, **Lyc, Merc,** *Phos*, *Puls*, *Rhus*, Sang, **Sep, Sil,** *Sulf*, **Tub; wet** weather<: **Ars,** Bell, Bry, **Calc,** *Carb-v*, Hep, *Iod*, Ipec, *Lyc*, *Merc*, **Nat-s,** Phos, *Puls*, **Rhus,** Seneg, Sep, **Sil,** *Sulf*, **Tub; feeling** in bloodvessels: **Acon,** Ant-t, **Ars,** Lyc, **Rhus.**

Collapse: Ars, Carb-v, Iod, Merc, *Phos*, sudden: **Ars,** Phos, a. vomiting: **Ars,** Lob.

Cynosis: Acon, *Ant-t*, *Ars*, *Bell*, Bry, Calc, **Carb-v,** Chel, Hep, *Ipec*, Lyc, Phos, Puls, *Rhus*, Seneg, Sil, Sulf.

Dry weather: <: Ars, *Bry*, ~~Carb-v~~, **Hep**, Phos, *Sep*, Sil, Sulf.

Dwarfish subjects: *Calc*, Iod, Lyc, Merc, *Sil*, **Sulf.**

Eating: B.: Acon, Ars, Bell, Bry, *Calc*, Carb-v, *Chel*, Hep, **Iod,** Merc, **Phos,** *Puls*, *Rhus*, Seneg, Sep, Sil, *Sulf*; **d.:** Ant-t, Ars, Bell, *Bry*, *Calc*, **Carb-v,** *Hep*, Iod, *Lyc*, Merc, *Phos*, *Puls*, Rhus, *Sep*, Sil, **Sulf; a.:** Acon, Ant-t, **Ars,** *Bell*, **Bry, Calc,** *Carb-v*, *Chel*, Ferr-p, Hep, Iod, Ipec, **Lyc,** Merc, Nat-s, **Phos, Puls,** *Rhus*, Sang, *Seneg*, **Sep, Sil, Sulf, >:** Acon, Ars, *Bry*, Calc, *Chel*, *Hep*, **Iod,** Merc, **Phos,** *Puls*, Rhus, **Sep,** Sil; to **satiety:** *Calc*, Carb-v, **Lyc, Puls,** Sep, Sil, *Sulf*.

Emaciated subjects: Ant-t, **Ars,** *Bry*, **Calc,** *Carb-v*, *Chel*, *Hep*, **Iod,** *Ipec*, **Lyc,** *Merc*, *Nat-s*, **Phos,** *Puls*, Sep, **Sil, Sulf, Tub; children: Ars, Calc,** *Carb-v*, **Iod,** *Lyc*, *Phos*, *Puls*, *Sep*, **Sil,** *Sulf*; **aged: Iod, Lyc;** pining **boys: Lyc, Tub.**

Exertion, physical, <: Acon, *Ant-t*, **Ars, Bry, Calc,** *Carb-v*, *Chel*, Ferr-p, *Hep*, **Iod,** Ipec, *Lob*, *Lyc*, *Merc*, *Phos*, *Puls*, **Rhus,** *Sang*, **Sep,** *Sil*, **Sulf,** *Tub*; >: **Rhus, Sep,** Sil.

Faintness: Morning: **Ars,** *Carb-v*, Puls, *Sang*, **Sulf,** on rising: **Bry, Carb-v,** *Iod*, Sep, **11** a. m.: **Sulf; chill,** d.: Ars, **Sep;** close **room:** Acon, Ipec, **Puls;** crowded room: Ars, *Lyc*, *Phos*, **Puls,** Sulf; **exertion:** *Ars*, Calc, *Carb-v*, **Sep,** Sulf; **fever,** d.: *Acon*, Bell, *Phos*, **Sep; frequent: Ars,** *Phos*, **Sulf; fright,** a.: **Acon;** with **heat** then coldness: [**Sep**]; **menses,** d.: Calc, *Puls*, **Sep,** Sulf; **motion: Ars; rising** from bed: Acon, **Bry,** *Carb-v*, Iod, Rhus, Sep; **sitting** up: **Acon, Bry,** Carb-v, *Ipec*, Sulf, Verat-v; **urination,** a.: **Acon; vomiting,** a.: **Ars; waking: Carb-v; warm** room: *Acon*, *Ipec*, Lyc, **Puls, Sep.**

Foggy weather: <: Bry, **Rhus,** Sep, *Sil*, Sulf.

Food: Beans and peas: <: Ars, **Bry,** *Calc*, Carb-v, **Lyc,** Puls, Sep, Sil; **bread <: Bry,** Merc, Phos, **Puls,** *Rhus*, *Sep*, *Sulf*, and butter <: Phos, **Puls,** *Sep*, Sulf; **butter <:** Acon, Ant-t, *Ars*, Bell, **Carb-v,** Hep, Ipec, *Phos*, **Puls,** *Sep*, Sulf; cold **drinks <:**

Ars, *Bell*, Calc, *Carb-v*, *Chel*, *Lyc*, Merc, Puls, **Rhus,** *Sil*, *Sulf*, >: *Ant-t*, Ars, **Bry,** Calc, **Phos,** *Puls*, **Sep;** cold **food**<: **Ars,** *Bry*, Calc, *Carb-v*, Chel, *Hep*, **Lyc,** *Merc*, *Nat-s*, *Puls*, **Rhus,** *Sep*, **Sil,** *Sulf*; **Flatulent** food<: Ars, **Bry,** Calc, Carb-v, **Lyc,** Puls, Sep, Sil; **fruit<:** Acon, Ant-t, **Ars, Bry,** Calc, *Carb-v*, *Ipec*, *Lyc*, **Nat-s,** Phos, **Puls,** *Sep*; **milk<:** Ant-t, *Ars*, *Bry*, **Calc,** *Carb-v*, *Chel*, *Lyc*, *Nat-s*, *Phos*, *Puls*, Rhus, **Sep,** Sil, **Sulf; onions<: Lyc,** *Puls*; **rich** food<: *Bry*, **Carb-v,** *Ipec*, *Nat-s*, Phos, **Puls,** *Sep*; **Sight** of,<: Ant-t, *Lyc*, **Sulf; veal**<: Ars, *Calc*, **Ipec,** *Sep*, Sulf; **vegetables** (green):<: Ars, *Bry*, Lyc, **Nat-s; warm** drinks>: **Ars,** *Bry*, *Chel*, *Lyc*, **Rhus,** *Sulf*; warm food<: Acon, Ant-t, *Bell*, **Bry,** Calc, *Carb-v*, Merc, **Phos, Puls,** *Rhus*, Sep, Sil, Sulf.

Heat, lack of vital: **Ars, Calc,** *Carb-v*, *Chel*, **Hep,** *Ipec*, *Lyc*, *Merc*, **Phos, Rhus,** *Sep*, **Sil,** *Sulf*, *Tub*.

Heated, becoming: Acon, *Bell*, **Bry,** *Carb-v*, Hep, **Iod,** Ipec, Merc, *Phos*, **Puls,** *Sep*, **Sil.**

Irritability, excessive physical: Acon, *Ant-t*, *Ars*, **Bell,** Bry, Hep, **Merc,** *Phos*, *Puls*, Rhus, Sep, **Sil,** Sulf; **lack** of: Ant-t, *Ars*, Bry, **Calc, Carb-v,** *Iod*, *Ipec*, *Lyc*, Phos, Rhus, Seneg, *Sep*, *Sulf*.

Jar, stepping:<: *Acon*, Ars, **Bell, Bry,** *Calc*, Chel, *Hep*, *Lyc*, Merc, *Phos*, *Puls*, **Rhus,** Seneg, *Sep*, **Sil,** *Sulf*.

Lassitude: Acon, *Ant-t*, *Ars*, *Bell*, Bry, **Calc,** *Carb-v*, *Chel*, Ferr-p, *Hep*, Iod, Ipec, *Lob*, *Lyc*, *Merc*, *Phos*, Puls, *Rhus*, **Sang,** *Seneg*, *Sep*, **Sil,** *Sulf*.

Lean people: Bry, *Iod*, *Lyc*, *Phos*, Sep, *Sil*, **Sulf,** Tub.

Lie down, inclined to: **Acon,** Ant-t, **Ars,** *Bell*, Bry, *Calc*, *Carb-v*, *Chel*, Ferr-p, Ipec, *Lyc*, Merc, *Phos*, *Puls*, *Rhus*, *Sep*, **Sil,** *Sulf*.

Lying:<: *Acon*, *Ant-t*, **Ars,** *Bell*, *Bry*, Calc, Carb-v, Chel, Ferr-p, Hep, Iod, Ipec, **Lyc,** Merc, **Nat-s, Phos, Puls, Rhus, Sang,** Seneg, *Sep*, *Sulf*; >: Acon, Ant-t, Ars, **Bell, Bry, Calc,** *Carb-v*, Chel, Hep, Iod, Ipec, Lyc, Merc, Phos, Rhus, Seneg, Sep, *Sulf*; **a.:<:** Acon Ant-t, **Ars,** Bell, Bry, Calc, Carb-v, Chel, Hep, Ipec,

Lyc, Merc, Phos, **Puls, Rhus,** Seneg, *Sep*, Sil, *Sulf*,>: Acon, Ant-t, **Ars,** *Bell*, **Bry, Calc,** *Carb-v*, Chel, *Hep*, *Iod*, Ipec, Lyc, *Merc*, Phos, **Puls,** Rhus, *Sep*, Sil, *Sulf*; on **abdomen:>:** Ars, **Bell,** Bry, Calc, *Chel*, *Phos*, Rhus, Sep; on **back:<:** Acon, *Ars*, Bell, Bry, Calc, *Iod*, Merc, *Nat-s*, **Phos,** *Rhus*, *Sep*, *Sil*, *Sulf*,>: *Acon*, Bell, **Bry, Calc,** Ipec, *Lyc*, Merc, *Nat-s*, *Phos*, **Puls, Rhus,** *Sang*, *Seneg*, Sep, Sil, Sulf; in **bed:<:** Acon, *Ant-t*, *Ars*, Bell, *Bry*, Calc, Carb-v, Chel, Hep, **Iod, Lyc, Merc, Phos, Puls,** *Rhus*, **Sang, Sep, Sil, Sulf,**>: *Acon*, Ant-t, *Ars*, Bell, **Bry,** Calc, Carb-v, Chel, **Hep,** Iod, Ipec, *Lyc*, Merc, Phos, Puls, *Rhus*, Sep, *Sil*, Sulf; on **sides:**<: **Acon,** Bell, **Bry, Calc,** *Ipec*, **Lyc,** *Merc*, *Nat-s*, *Phos*, *Puls*, **Rhus,** *Seneg*, Sep, *Sil*, *Sulf*,>: Acon, Ars, Bell, Bry, Iod, *Phos*, Rhus, *Sep*, Sulf; **r.** side:<: Acon, Bry, Ipec, Lyc, **Merc,** *Phos*, Seneg, Sulf; **l.** side:<: *Acon*, Ant-t, Bell, Bry, Ipec, Lyc, Merc, *Nat-s*, **Phos, Puls,** Rhus, Seneg, *Sep*, Sil, *Sulf*; **painful** side:<: *Acon*, *Ars*, *Bell*, Bry, Calc, Carb-v, **Hep, Iod,** *Lyc*, *Merc*, *Phos*, Puls, *Rhus*, Sep, **Sil,>:** Bell, **Bry,** *Calc*, Carb-v, Lyc, *Puls*, Rhus, *Sep*, Sulf; **painless** side:<: Bell, **Bry,** *Calc*, Carb-v, Chel, Lyc, Phos, **Puls,** *Rhus*, *Sep*.

Magnetism:>: Acon, *Bell*, *Calc*, Iod, **Phos,** Sep, *Sil*, Sulf.

Measles, a.: *Bell*, Bry, **Carb-v, Puls,** *Rhus*, *Sulf*.

Motion:<: *Acon*, Ant-t, *Ars*, **Bell, Bry,** Calc, *Carb-v*, **Chel,** *Hep*, *Iod*, *Ipec*, **Merc,** *Nat-s*, *Phos*, Puls, *Sang*, Seneg, *Sep*, **Sil, Sulf;>:** *Acon*, Ant-t, *Ars*, Calc, Carb-v, Ferr-p, Hep, Lob, **Lyc,** *Nat-s*, **Puls, Rhus,** Seneg, *Sep*, **Sulf,** *Tub*; < at **beginning:** Ant-t Calc, *Carb-v*, **Lyc,** *Phos*, **Puls, Rhus,** *Sil*; **a.,** <: **Ars,** *Carb-v*, Iod, Merc, Phos, **Puls, Rhus,** Sep; of **affected** parts: *Acon*, *Ant-t*, *Ars*, *Bell*, **Bry,** Chel, Hep, Iod, *Merc*, *Phos*, *Puls*, **Rhus,** *Sang*, Sep, *Sil*, *Sulf*,>: Acon, *Ars*, Calc, *Lyc*, **Puls, Rhus,** *Sep*, **Sulf; aversion** to: **Acon,** Ant-t, **Ars, Bell, Bry, Calc,** *Carb-v*, *Chel*, Ipec, *Lyc*, Merc, Phos, Puls, *Sang*, Sep, **Sil, Sulf; continued:>:** Bry, Carb-v, *Lyc*, **Puls, Rhus,** Sep, *Sil*.

Mucus secretions increased: Acon, Ant-t, *Ars*, *Bell*, Bry, **Calc**, **Carb-v**, Chel, *Hep*, **Iod**, *Ipec*, **Lyc**, **Merc**, **Phos**, **Puls**, *Rhus*, *Seneg*, *Sep*, *Sil*, **Sulf.**

Obese subjects: Bry, **Calc**, Iod, Ipec, *Lyc*, Merc, *Puls*, Seneg, Sep, Sil, *Sulf*.

Old people: *Acon*, Ant-t, *Ars*, Bry, *Carb-v*, *Iod*, **Lyc**, *Seneg*, Sulf.

PAIN:> and < suddenly: Bell; **biting:** Carb-v, Sulf; **boring:** Bell, Puls; **burning:** Ars, Bry, Carb-v, Merc, Phos, Rhus, Sep, Sil, Sulf, ext.: Acon, Ars, Bell, Bry, Merc, Phos, Puls, Rhus, Sang, Sep, Sulf, in bloodvessels: Ars, Rhus; **constricting** ext.: Puls; **cutting** ext.: Bell, Calc, int,: Bell, Calc, Lyc, Merc, Puls, Sil, Sulf; **drawing:** Carb-v, Chel, **gnawing:** Merc, int.: Puls, Sep; **jerking** ext.: Calc, Puls, Rhus, int.: Bell, Puls, Sil, Sulf; **paralytic:** Bell: **pinching:** Bell, int.: Calc, Chel, Lyc; **pressing** ext.: Phos, Puls, Rhus, Sep, Sil, Sulf, int.: Ars, Bell, Calc, Carb-v, Lyc, Phos, Puls, Rhus, Sang, Seneg, Sep, Sil, Sulf, as from a load: Acon, Bell, Bry, Ipec, Phos, Rhus, Sep, Sulf, together: Sulf, within outward: Bry, Puls,Sulf; **scraped,** as if: Puls, Sulf; **sore,** bruised: Rhus, Sil, ext.: Bell, Hep, Rhus, Sil, Sulf, int.: Puls; **splinter-like:** Hep; **stitching** ext.: Bell, Bry, Calc, Merc, Puls, Rhus, Sulf, int.: Bry, Chel, Merc, Phos, Puls, Sep, Sil, burning: Ars, downward: Carb-v, Rhus, outward: Chel, Merc, Sulf, transversely: Bell, upward: Bell, Sep; **tearing** ext.: Acon, Bell, Bry, Lyc, Nat-s, Puls, Sep, Sil, Sulf, int.: Bell, Bry, Carb-v, Lyc, Merc, Puls, Sep, Sil, Sulf, tearing away: Rhus, downward: Bell, Lyc, Rhus, Sulf, upward: Bell, Sep, Sil; **twisting:** Sil; **ulcerative** ext.: Bry, Puls, Rhus, Sil, int.: Puls, Sil; **wandering:** Puls.

Perspiration does not>: *Acon*, *Ant-t*, **Ars**, Bell, *Calc*, Carb-v, Chel, *Hep*, *Ipec*, Lyc, **Merc**, *Phos*, *Puls*, **Rhus**, **Sep**, **Sulf**, *Verat-v*,>: *Ars*, **Bry**, Calc, Lyc, Rhus, **a.:<:** Ars, Bell, Bry, *Calc*, Carb-v, Iod, Lyc, *Merc*, *Phos*, *Puls*, **Sep**, Sil, *Sulf*,>: *Acon*, Ant-t, *Ars*, Bell, *Bry*, Chel, *Hep*, Ipec, Lyc, Puls,

Rhus, *Sulf*; **suppression** of: Acon, Ars, **Bell,** *Bry,* **Calc,** *Carb-v, Hep,* Iod, Ipec, *Lyc, Merc, Nat-s, Phos,* Puls, **Rhus,** Seneg, **Sep, Sil, Sulf.**

Plethoric subjects: *Acon, Ars,* **Bell, Bry, Calc,** *Carb-v,* Chel, Ferr-p, Hep, Iod, Ipec, **Lyc,** *Merc,* **Phos,** *Puls, Rhus,* Seneg, **Sep, Sil, Sulf.**

Pressure:<: Acon, *Ars,* Bell, *Bry,* Calc, *Carb-v, Chel,* **Hep, Iod,** Ipec, **Lyc,** *Merc, Nat-s,* Phos, Puls, Rhus, Seneg, Sep, **Sil,** Sulf;**>**: Acon, Ars, Bell, **Bry,** Calc, *Chel,* Ipec, Merc, *Nat-s,* Phos, **Puls,** *Rhus,* Sang, *Sep,* **Sil,** Sulf; on **painless** side:<: Bell, **Bry,** *Calc,* Carb-v, Lyc, **Puls,** *Rhus, Sep.*

Pulse: Abnormal: **Acon,** *Ant-t,* **Ars, Bell,** *Bry,* Calc, *Carb-v,* Chel, *Hep,* **Iod,** Ipec, Lyc, *Merc,* **Phos,** Puls, **Rhus,** Seneg, *Sep,* **Sil,** *Sulf*; **frequent: Acon,** *Ant-t,* **Ars, Bell, Bry,** Calc, Carb-v, Chel, **Ferr-p,** Hep, **Iod,** Ipec, Lob, Lyc, **Merc,** *Nat-s,* **Phos,** *Puls,* **Rhus,** *Sang,* Seneg, *Sep,* **Sil, Sulf, Verat-v,** a. eating: *Iod,* **Lyc,** *Phos, Puls,* Rhus, *Sulf,* a. vexation: Acon, **Sep,** and small: **Acon, Ars,** Bell, Bry, *Iod,* Lob, Lyc, Phos, Puls, Rhus, **Sil; full: Acon, Ant-t,** Ars, **Bell, Bry, Chel,** Ferr-p, *Hep,* Iod, Lyc, *Merc, Phos,* Rhus, Sang, Seneg, *Sep, Sil, Sulf, Verat-v*; **hard: Acon,** *Ant-t,* Ars, **Bell, Bry, Chel,** *Hep,* Iod, Lyc, *Merc, Phos,* Seneg, *Sep, Sil, Sulf,* Verat-v; **imperceptible: Acon,** Ant-t, *Ars,* Bell, **Carb-v,** Chel, *Ipec, Merc,* Phos, Puls, Rhus, **Sil,** Sulf, almost: **Acon,** Ant-t, *Ars,* Bell, *Ipec, Merc,* Phos, *Puls, Rhus,* Seneg; **intermittent:** *Acon, Ars,* Bell, *Bry, Carb-v, Hep, Iod,* Lob, **Merc,** Phos, *Rhus, Sep, Sulf,* Verat-v; **irregular: Acon,** Ant-t, **Ars,** Bell, *Bry,* Calc, Carb-v, Chel, Iod, Lob, *Merc, Phos, Rhus, Sang,* Seneg, *Sep, Sil, Sulf,* **Verat-v,** and slow: Acon, Ars, Bell, Chel, Iod, Lob, Rhus, Seneg, **Verat-v, slow:** *Acon, Ant-t,* Ars, *Bell, Chel,* Hep, Iod, *Lob,* Merc, Phos, Puls, Rhus, *Sang,* **Sep,** Sil, *Verat-v*; **small: Acon,** *Ant-t,* **Ars,** *Bell,* Bry, Calc, **Carb-v,** *Iod,* Ipec, *Lob,* Lyc, *Merc, Phos,* Puls, Rhus, Seneg, **Sil,** *Sulf*; **soft:** *Acon,* **Ant-t,** *Ars,* Bell, Bry, **Carb-v,** Hep, Iod, Ipec, *Lob,* Lyc, *Merc, Phos,* Puls, Rhus, *Sang,* Seneg, Sil, *Verat-v*; **tremulous:** Acon,

Ant-t, *Ars*, *Bell*, **Calc,** Iod, Merc, Phos, *Rhus*, *Sep*; **weak:** Acon, **Ant-t, Ars,** Bell, Bry, **Carb-v,** *Iod*, *Ipec*, Lob, *Merc*, *Phos*, *Puls*, *Rhus*, *Sang*, Seneg, Sep, *Verat-v*.

Reaction, lack of: Ant-t, *Ars*, Bry, **Calc, Carb-v,** *Iod*, *Ipec*, *Lyc*, *Merc*, *Phos*, Seneg, *Sep*, **Sulf.**

Rising:<: Acon, *Ant-t*, *Ars*, **Bell, Bry,** *Chel*, Hep, **Lyc,** Merc, *Phos*, *Puls*, **Rhus,** *Sang*, Seneg, Sep, **Sil, Sulf,** Verat-v;>: Acon, *Ant-t*, **Ars,** Bell, Bry, **Calc,** Carb-v, Chel, Hep, *Lyc*, Merc, Phos, Puls, Rhus, **Sep,** *Sil*, Sulf.

Rubbing:<: Ars, Calc, Chel, Merc, **Puls,** Seneg, **Sep,** *Sil*, **Sulf;**>: Acon, Ant-t, *Ars*, Bell, Bry, **Calc,** Chel, Hep, *Merc*, **Phos,** Rhus, Seneg, *Sulf*.

Scarlet fever, a.: **Bell,** *Bry*, *Calc*, *Carb-v*, *Hep*, Lyc, *Merc*, Phos, Rhus, *Sulf*.

Sensitive: Ext.: *Acon*, Ant-t, Ars, **Bell,** Bry, Calc, Carb-v, Ferr-p, *Hep*, Ipec, Lyc, *Merc*, **Phos, Puls,** *Rhus*, *Seneg*, *Sep*, **Sil,** *Sulf*; **int.:** Acon, Ant-t, *Ars*, *Bell*, *Bry*, *Calc*, Carb-v, **Hep,** *Iod*, Ipec, Merc, **Phos,** Puls, Rhus, Seneg, Sep, **Sil,** Sulf; to **pain:** *Acon*, Ant-t, *Ars*, *Bell*, *Bry*, Calc, Carb-v, Ferr-p, **Hep,** Iod, Ipec, **Lyc,** Merc, **Phos,** *Rhus*, Seneg, **Sep, Sil,** Sulf, *Tub*.

Sitting:<: Acon, Ant-t, **Ars,** Bell, *Bry*, Calc, Carb-v, Chel, Hep, Iod, Ipec, **Lyc,** *Merc*, **Phos, Puls, Rhus,** *Seneg*, **Sep,** Sil, **Sulf;>:** *Acon*, *Ant-t*, Ars, Calc, Carb-v, Chel, Hep, Iod, Ipec, *Merc*, Phos, *Puls*, *Sil*, Sulf; must sit up in bed with knees drawn up, rests head and arms on knees: [**Ars**].

Sleep: B.:<: Acon, **Ars,** *Bell*, **Bry, Calc, Carb-v,** Chel, *Hep*, Ipec, *Lyc*, **Merc, Phos, Puls, Rhus,** Seneg, **Sep,** *Sil*, **Sulf;** at **beginning** of: **Ars, Bell, Bry,** *Calc*, *Carb-v*, Hep, Ipec, *Lyc*, *Merc*, *Phos*, **Puls,** *Rhus*, **Sep,** Sil, *Sulf*; **d.:** <: *Acon*, *Ant-t*, **Ars, Bell, Bry,** Calc, *Chel*, **Hep,** Ipec, *Lyc*, **Merc,** *Phos*, *Puls*, Rhus, Seneg, *Sep*, **Sil, Sulf; a.:** <: *Acon*, *Ars*, Bell, Bry, Calc, *Carb-v*, *Chel*, *Hep*, *Lyc*, *Phos*, *Puls*, Rhus, *Sep*, **Sulf,**>: Acon, *Ars*, Bry, Calc, Ipec, *Merc*, **Phos,** Puls, Sang, *Sep*.

Snow-air:<: *Calc*, *Lyc*, Merc, *Phos*, *Puls*, *Rhus*, **Sep,** *Sil*, *Sulf*.

Standing:<: Acon, Ars, *Bell*, *Bry*, *Calc*, Carb-v, Chel, Ferr-p, Hep, Merc, Phos, **Puls,** *Rhus*, **Sep,** *Sil*, **Sulf,** *Tub*; **>:** Ant-t, **Ars, Bell,** Bry, Calc, Carb-v, Chel, Hep, *Iod*, Ipec, Merc, *Phos*.

Stone-cutters: Calc, Ipec, *Lyc*, *Puls*, **Sil,** Sulf.

Stretching: Acon, Ant-t, **Ars,** *Bell*, *Calc*, *Carb-v*, Chel, Hep, Lob, *Merc*, Nat-s, *Phos*, **Puls, Rhus,** *Sep*, Sil, Sulf; b. urination: [**Puls**].

Sycotic subjects: Ant-t, Bry, *Calc*, Carb-v, Hep, *Iod*, *Lyc*, Merc, **Nat-s,** Puls, **Sep,** *Sil*, *Sulf*.

Syphilitic subjects: *Ars*, Carb-v, *Hep*, *Iod*, **Merc,** *Phos*, **Sil,** *Sulf*.

Touch:<: *Acon*, *Ant-t*, *Ars*, **Bell, Bry,** Calc, *Carb-v*, *Chel*, **Hep,** *Iod*, Ipec, **Lyc,** *Merc*, *Phos*, *Puls*, **Rhus,** *Sang*, *Seneg*, **Sep, Sil, Sulf; slight:<:** Ars, **Bell, Merc,** *Phos*.

Touching cold things:<: Calc, **Hep,** *Merc*, **Rhus, Sil.**

Uncovering:<: *Acon*, **Ars,** *Bell*, *Bry*, **Hep, Lyc,** *Merc*, *Phos*, Puls, **Rhus,** Sep, **Sil;** single parts:<: *Bry*, **Hep, Rhus, Sil.**

Undressing:<: Ars, Calc, Hep, Nat-s, *Puls*, **Rhus,** Sep, *Sil*.

Vaccination, a.: *Ars*, Hep, **Sil, Sulf.**

Vomiting:<: Acon, *Ant-t*, **Ars,** Bell, *Bry*, *Calc*, Iod, **Ipec,** *Lyc*, *Phos*, **Puls,** *Sep*, Sil, **Sulf.**

Waking: Acon, Ant-t, **Ars,** Bell, Bry, **Calc,** *Chel*, **Hep,** *Ipec*, *Lyc*, *Merc*, **Phos, Puls,** *Rhus*, *Sang*, Seneg, **Sep,** *Sil*, **Sulf; >:** *Ars*, Bry, Calc, Ipec, **Phos,** Puls, **Sep.**

Warm:< Acon, *Ant-t*, Bell, *Bry*, Carb-v, **Iod,** *Ipec*, *Lyc*, *Merc*, *Nat-s*, *Phos*, **Puls,** *Seneg*, *Sulf*; air:<: *Ant-t*, *Bry*, Calc, **Iod,** *Ipec*, *Lyc*, **Merc,** *Nat-s*, *Phos*, **Puls,** *Seneg*, *Sulf*; **bed:<:** *Ant-t*, *Bry*, Calc,

Carb-v, *Iod*, *Ipec*, *Lyc*, **Merc**, Phos, **Puls**, *Seneg*, **Sulf**, >: **Ars**, Bell, **Bry**, **Hep**, **Lyc**, *Phos*, **Rhus**, *Sep*, **Sil**, Sulf, **Tub**; **room**: <: Acon, Ant-t, Bell, *Bry*, Calc, *Carb-v*, **Iod**, *Ipec*, **Lyc**, Merc, *Nat-s*, Phos, **Puls**, **Seneg**, **Sulf**, *Tub*; **stove**: >: Acon, **Ars**, Bell, **Hep**, **Rhus**, **Sil**, Sulf; wet **weather**: <: **Carb-v**, *Iod*, **Nat-s**, *Sil*; **wraps**: <: *Acon*, *Bry*, *Calc*, Carb-v, **Iod**, **Lyc**, Merc, Phos, **Puls**, Rhus, *Seneg*, Sep, **Sulf**.

Weakness: *Acon*, **Ant-t**, **Ars**, Bell, *Bry*, **Calc**, *Carb-v*, **Chel**, Ferr-p, **Hep**, **Iod**, *Ipec*, Lob, *Lyc*, **Merc**, **Nat-s**, **Phos**, *Puls*, **Rhus**, *Sang*, *Seneg*, **Sep**, **Sil**, **Sulf**, **Tub**, Verat-v; **morning**: **Ars**, Bell, *Bry*, *Calc*, *Carb-v*, Chel; *Iod*, **Lyc**, *Merc*, *Nat-s*, *Phos*, *Puls*, *Rhus*, Sang, **Sep**, *Sil*, *Sulf*, in bed: *Carb-v*, Hep, Phos, **Puls**, *Sil*, lying: [**Puls**], rising: **Bry**, Hep, *Lyc*, Phos, *Sep*, *Sil*, Sulf; **forenoon**: Acon, Ant-t, **Bry**, Carb-v, *Lyc*, Sep; **afternoon**: Acon, Bell, *Bry*, Lyc, Nat-s, Rhus, Sang, *Sil*, **Sulf**; **eating**, a.: **Ars**, Hep, *Lyc*, Phos, Rhus, Sang, *Sil*, Sulf; **exertion**, least: Acon, **Ars**, **Bry**, **Calc**, *Carb-v*, *Lyc*, *Merc*, **Phos**, **Rhus** *Sep*, *Sulf*; **fever**, d.: Acon, Ant-t, **Ars**, *Bry*, Carb-v, Lyc, **Phos**, *Puls*, *Rhus*, Sulf: **hunger**, from: **Iod**, *Phos*, **Sulf**; mental **exertion**: Ars, *Bell*, **Calc**, *Lyc*, **Puls**, Sep, Sil, *Sulf*; **motion**: **Ars**, Bry, Merc, *Phos*, Sulf; **nervous**: Acon, Ars, *Bell*, Bry, *Calc*, Carb-v, Hep, *Iod*, Lyc, *Merc*, **Phos**, **Puls**, Rhus, **Sep**, **Sil**, *Sulf*; **pain**, from: **Ars**, Carb-v, *Rhus*; **paralytic**: **Ars**, Bell, Bry, *Calc*, Carb-v, Chel, *Merc*, **Phos**, *Puls*, *Rhus*, Sil, slides down in bed: *Ars*, Carb-v, **Phos**, *Rhus*; **sweat**, from: Acon, *Ars*, **Bry**, *Calc*, Carb-v, Ferr-p, **Iod**, Lyc, **Merc**, **Phos**, Puls, **Sep**, *Sil*, *Sulf*, **Tub**, *Verat-v*, night: Ars, Bry, *Merc*, **Tub**; **rapid**: **Ars**, *Sep*; **rising**: **Ars**, **Bry**, Lyc, *Rhus*; **sitting**: *Ars*, Bry, Chel, *Lyc*, **Rhus**, *Sulf*; **stool**, a.: Ant-t, **Ars**, *Calc*, *Carb-v*, *Iod*, Ipec, *Lyc*, **Merc**, **Nat-s**, *Phos*, *Sep*, *Sulf*, **tremulous**: *Ars*, Carb-v, Hep, Lyc, *Phos*, *Puls*, *Sep*; **sudden**: Acon, **Ars**, Calc, *Carb-v*, *Hep*, *Ipec*, Lyc, *Phos*, **Sep**; **talking**: *Calc*, Iod, Sep, Sil, **Sulf**; **waking**: Bell, Bry, Chel, Ferr-p, Lyc, **Puls**, Rhus, Sang, *Sep*, Sulf; warm **room**: *Iod*, **Puls**.

Weariness: Morning: *Ars*, *Carb-v*, **Sep,** *Sulf*; eating, a.: **Ars,** *Rhus*, Sang.

Wet: Applications: *Bell*, Bry, **Calc,** Carb-v, *Lyc*, *Merc*, Phos, Puls, **Rhus,** *Sep*, Sil, **Sulf; getting:** Ars, *Bell*, *Bry*, **Calc,** Carb-v, *Hep*, *Ipec*, *Lyc*, Phos, **Puls, Rhus, Sep,** Sulf, feet: Merc, *Phos*, **Puls,** *Rhus*, *Sep*, **Sil,** head: **Bell,** *Puls*, d. sweat: *Acon*, Calc, **Rhus,** *Sep*; **weather:** <: *Ant-t*, **Ars,** Bell, Bry, **Calc,** *Carb-v*, *Hep*, *Iod*, Ipec, *Lyc*, *Merc*, **Nat-s,** Phos, **Puls, Rhus,** Sang, Seneg, *Sep*, *Sil*, *Sulf*, *Tub*.

Wind: *Acon*, *Ars*, *Bell*, Bry, Calc, Carb-v, **Lyc, Phos, Puls,** Sulf; **cold:** *Acon*, *Ars*, **Bell,** *Bry*, Carb-v, **Hep,** Ipec, *Sep*, *Sil*.

Winter: *Acon*, *Ars*, *Bell*, *Bry*, *Calc*, Carb-v, *Hep*, Ipec, Lyc, *Merc*, *Phos*, Puls, **Rhus,** *Sep*, *Sil*, Sulf.

The End